Occupational Therapy

WHAT IT IS & HOW IT WORKS

Occupational Therapy

WHAT IT IS & HOW IT WORKS

WILLIAM MATTHEW MARCIL
PhD, MS, OTR/L, FAOTA

THOMSON
★
DELMAR LEARNING

Australia Brazil Canada Mexico Singapore Spain United Kingdom United States

THOMSON

DELMAR LEARNING

Occupational Therapy: What It Is and How It Works
by William Matthew Marcil, PhD, MS, OTR/L, FAOTA

Vice President, Health Care Business Unit:
William Brottmiller

Director of Learning Solutions:
Matthew Kane

Senior Acquisitions Editor:
Sherry Dickinson

Product Manager:
Juliet Steiner

Editorial Assistant:
Angela Doolin

Marketing Director:
Jennifer McAvey

Marketing Manager:
Christopher Manion

Marketing Coordinator:
Danielle Pacella

Production Director:
Carolyn Miller

Production Manager:
Barbara A. Bullock

Content Project Manager:
Jessica McNavich

Library of Congress Cataloging-in-Publication Data
Marcil, William Matthew.
  Occupational therapy : what it is and how it works / William Matthew Marcil.
     p. cm.
  Includes bibliographical references and index.
  1. Occupational therapy.
I. Title.
  RC487.M37 2007
  616.89'165—dc22
           2006018987
ISBN-13: 978-1-4180-1285-4
ISBN-10: 1-4180-1285-8

NOTICE TO THE READER

DEDICATION

To my parents
John and Marilyn Marcil
Who gave me life

To my brothers and sisters
John, Lynn, Holly, and Dan
Who shaped my life

To my dear friend and mentor
Kent Nelson Tigges, MS, OTR, FAOTA, FHIH (in memoriam)
Who changed my life

To Loryn, Courtney, Natalie, and Meredith
Who share my life

ABOUT THE AUTHOR

William Matthew Marcil, Ph.D., MS, OTR/L, FAOTA, has been an occupational therapy practitioner since 1978 and has worked in a variety of health care settings throughout his career. A native of Albany, New York, Dr. Marcil is a staunch proponent of occupational therapy and has promoted the profession through numerous articles, books, book chapters, and videos. Additionally, he has presented lectures and workshops throughout the United States and across the world, including Australia, Canada, Guam, and New Zealand. Dr. Marcil is the director of the Occupational Therapy Assistant Program at Tidewater Community College in Virginia Beach, Virginia. He lives in Virginia Beach with his wife, Loryn, three daughters, Courtney, Natalie, and Meredith, three dogs, six cats, and numerous other flora and fauna.

CONTENTS

Part I: Occupational Therapy: What It Is

Part II: Occupational Therapy: How It Works

Chapter 6: How Does Occupational Therapy Fit Into the Health Care Team?

Chapter 7: The Occupational Therapy Process

PREFACE

Occupational therapy is perhaps the least known, most misunderstood, and most overlooked of all the health care professions. Although the profession has been in existence for almost 90 years, most people haven't the faintest idea of what occupational therapy is or how it works. Occupational therapy as important a health profession as it is—has been frequently overshadowed by its peers, including nursing, physical therapy, and speech therapy, to name a few.

The goal of this book is not only to make the reader aware of what occupational therapy is and how it works, but also to demonstrate how vital it can be to the lives of those who may require its unique and important service.

This book has been written with three specific audiences in mind: those who may be interested in occupational therapy as a career, first-year occupational therapy students, and those who just wish to further their knowledge about the profession of occupational therapy.

This book is meant to be an introduction and an overview of the profession. It does not go into explicit detail. If you desire such detail, there are numerous other texts that will meet your needs.

Why I Wrote This Book

Most books on occupational therapy are written by and directed toward other occupational therapists and also, perhaps, occupational therapy (or occupational therapy assistant) students. I have found that presenting the profession in the traditional manner is similar to taking a boat into the middle of the ocean and jumping in, in order to learn how to swim; some people can do it, but most cannot.

Consider this book a means of getting your feet wet and gradually wading out into deeper water. If you get a little bit nervous, you can always come back to shore until you are ready to venture out for a safe and comfortable swim, even though your feet may no longer touch the bottom.

I believe that this is the first book of its kind on this topic. I have tried to make the reading interesting and, at times, humorous. I have also tried, as best I could, to stay away from difficult verbiage (oops). I mean, I have tried to use words that normal people—like yourselves—will understand. There will be times when some of these words are unavoidable; in these cases, I have tried to explain them as best I could.

Some parts of the book you will find extremely interesting, if not downright fascinating. Other parts may bore you to tears. I ask you to read everything in order to gain an understanding of what I consider to be a wonderful profession. The last chapter, "A Day in the Life of an Occupational Therapist," will pull everything together in a way that is very real and understandable.

Ultimately, I hope that you will enjoy this book and that it will give you unique insight into a wonderful, dynamic, and important profession that can truly make a difference in the lives of those in need of its unique offerings.

ACKNOWLEDGEMENTS

The process of writing a book is a Herculean task and typically involves the efforts of many more people than just the author. Although the onus of responsibility of this book has fallen on me, I would like to thank the following people for their input and assistance in the production of this book:

The Class of 2007, Tidewater Community College Occupational Therapy Assistant Program, for proofreading and blunt commentary: Jo Battle, Michelle Brackett, Ashlee Bucher, Ann Cronce, Cassandra Hawkins, Pamela L. Jones, Maria Lawrence, Monsurat Layeni, Louise Lerner, Holly Martin, Maureen McBride, Angela Miller, Natalie Phillips, Michele Spiering, Melissa Vaughan, Jennifer Warner, Lori Webber, Tedra White, and Amy Yourchisin.

Anne Hunter, for keeping my head screwed on straight and for finding all of those annoying little errors.

The really important people at Thomson Delmar Learning: Kalen Conerly (Kalen, Kalen, Kalen)—you walked into my office to sell me books and walked out with a new author! Kristy Kauffman, who, inadvertently, got this whole thing rolling by setting up a sales call. Juliet Steiner, for helping move the whole process along very smoothly and painlessly. Molly Belmont, for keeping tabs on me when necessary.

Vickie Schindler, Ph.D., OTR/L, FAOTA, for her long-time friendship and influence on my career.

Ann Burke, Ph.D., OTR/L, FAOTA, for her professional guidance, input, and proofreading skills.

The enduring memory and spirit of Kent Nelson Tigges, MS, OTR, FAOTA, FHIH, who, in life, was my mentor and my dearest friend. Although he is no longer part of this terrestrial world, his sage wisdom continues to guide my life and my practice and, I believe, helped me a great deal in the production of this book ("I know you're out there, you SOB!").

John Morea, for countless favors in terms of media advice and assistance, and for being a Buffalo Bills fan!

Mark Rubenstein, for helping me to maintain my sanity in a seemingly insane world. Mark, you are a hero in your own right!

My oldest daughters, Courtney (age 7) and Natalie (age 5), both of whom took turns helping me write the book by pressing the space bar after I typed each word. You both really helped speed things up!

Lawrence Page and Sergey Brin, for inventing Google™. I believe that Velcro® and duct tape were two of the greatest inventions of the 20th century and that Google™ is certainly one of the greatest inventions of the 21st century!

To the following people who, over the years, helped to forge and reshape my unusual sense of humor, which I believe is one of God's greatest gifts to humanity: my brothers, Danny and John Marcil, Jerry "Get" Bently, Joe Breslin, Ellen DeGeneres, Bill Engvall, Will Ferrel, Firesign Theater, Jeff Foxworthy, Professor Carl Hurley, Steve Martin, Monty Python's *Flying Circus, National Lampoon*, Dan Papandrea, the Reverend M. Alton Plummer, Brian Regan, Mark Rubenstein, and Steven Wright.

All of the professionals who have helped to shape my career and my professional life, some of whom I've never actually met.

Finally, to all of the people whom I have treated and had the honor to know: you are the people who have taught me the most about the good and the bad of life, and most of you have made my career a very enjoyable one.

What the Heck Is Occupational Therapy, Anyway?

In the summer of 1976, I was a 22-year-old aspiring rock star. I knew that my big break would come someday.

The Problem: When?

The economic recession made it difficult to find work at that time, but I knew that I needed to find something to pay the rent until my big break came.

The Problem: What?

The frustration of not finding a job finally led me to ponder continuing my education. It was late in the summer, and my prospects of being accepted into any program were slim. After being turned away from a number of colleges in my hometown of Albany, New York, I ventured into Maria College—a small, private college run by the Sisters of Mercy—to try my luck.

The school counselor talked with me, and reviewed my high school transcripts and limited transcripts from a local community college. She noted that I seemed to have done well in both art and science. She immediately followed this observation with a pronouncement: "You would do well in our occupational therapy assistant program."

"What the heck is occupational therapy?" I asked.

The counselor directed me to an adjoining building, where I descended into the basement classroom that was to become my home for the next two years. As I often tell people, I got into this profession by accident—the luckiest accident of my life. In reality, it was no accident. It was serendipity; that is, finding something quite valuable without having searched for it. By the way, the rock star thing didn't work out.

My original question—what is occupational therapy?—is one that I am asked by countless people on a weekly basis, and, after 26 years of practice, it is frustrating for me to constantly have to explain what I do. Mary Reilly (1962), one of the great philosophers of the profession, once stated that "Occupational therapy can be one of the greatest ideas of the twentieth century" (p. 2), and she was right. However, I would suggest that occupational therapy is one of the best-kept secrets of the 20th and, so far, the 21st century!

The Problem: Why?

I have pondered this question for many years and have concluded that so many people are unaware of what occupational therapy (OT) is because it is difficult to describe the profession in just a few words. Many therapists give long, drawn-out explanations that frequently leave the inquirers just as confused as they were before hearing the definition, if not more so.

In addition to often eclipsing *War and Peace* in length, the definitions usually vary based on the individual therapist's area of expertise and his frame of reference. I often tell people, only half jokingly, that if you were to gather 10 OTs in a room and ask them to each define OT, you would get 10 different definitions of the profession.

This inability to easily define what we do is, and has been, a problem for the profession, for what we do is extremely important. It is vital, however, that we let people know why we are important.

The Problem: How?

I ask my students, before they graduate, to define occupational therapy in 15 words or less; this usually turns out to be a difficult assignment for them. I have written this book to educate you, the reader, on exactly what comprises occupational therapy. When you are finished reading this book, I would like you to define occupational therapy in 15 words or less. See how you do.

This book is meant to be nothing more than an overview of the profession of occupational therapy, a profession that I personally care about very deeply. It is part text, part autobiography. For the most part, this book is my perception of the profession.

I have written this book using common language and simple terms to make the reading easy. However, there will be some terms that are seemingly clinical, dry, and boring. I have tried to keep these to a minimum, and I have tried to explain them in layman's terms whenever possible.

There may be some within my profession who object to my approach and style because of my humorous and sometimes irreverent perspective. To those people I say that I mean no disrespect for the profession; I merely want to present the information in a fun, lighthearted way in order to both keep and pique the reader's interest. I have a great love for this work, and my intent is to instill an interest in others in this fine and noble profession.

I must admit that I get very confused in terms of today's political correctness. When I was growing up, I learned to write in the masculine. I do not like to write in an ambiguous gender, so I have decided to intermix the pronouns he/she, his/her, etc. throughout the text rather than use cumbersome terminology. I hope that you, the reader, will find this acceptable.

I have written this book using commonly used vocabulary and have attempted to stay away from professional terms and buzzwords whenever possible. Unlike most introductory books to a profession, I have also used humor and personal anecdotes, where appropriate, to make my points. My personal belief is that effective learning must always involve the "F" word: FUN. If you have fun learning about something, you will remember it more easily.

My primary goal is to increase the general awareness of the occupational therapy profession. My secondary goal is to attract a number of new members to the profession. Like any other career, not everyone will like it or be well suited to it. I ask that you read this book and begin to ask yourself if this might be something that you would like to do. Before you begin your journey, ask yourself the following questions:

- Do I enjoy working with people?
- Do I enjoy helping people?
- Am I creative and inventive in my approach to problems?
- Am I flexible?
- Do I have a sense of humor?
- Do I get bored with drudgery and routine?
- Can I think *both* inside and outside of the box?

If you answered yes to any or all of these questions, I encourage you to read on. Occupational therapy may very well be your new career, or, perhaps, you will at least have a better understanding of the profession.

References

Reilly, M. (1962). Occupational therapy can be one of the greatest ideas of 20th-century medicine. *American Journal of Occupational Therapy. 16*(1), 2–9.

PART I

Occupational Therapy: What It Is

GIVE A MAN A FISH; YOU FEED HIM FOR TODAY.
TEACH A MAN TO FISH, AND YOU FEED HIM
FOR A LIFETIME.

- AUTHOR UNKNOWN

CHAPTER 1

What Is Occupational Therapy?

Chapter Goals

At the end of this chapter, the reader should:

- Be familiar with the official definition of occupational therapy.
- Have a functional definition of occupational therapy.
- Understand the importance of occupation for an optimally healthy lifestyle.
- Understand the multiple roles required to be an effective occupational therapist.

INTRODUCTION

This chapter will introduce the definition of occupational therapy and the skills required to become a good occupational therapist. The official definition of the American Occupational Therapy Association (AOTA) is presented as a baseline, and it is followed by information leading to a more user-friendly definition. The final part of this chapter will describe characteristics that are vital for an aspiring or practicing therapist.

Defining Occupational Therapy

The ability to define what you do in a succinct manner is an important skill to have. When two strangers meet for the first time—at a party, for instance—one of the first questions after "What's your name?" is inevitably "What do you do for a living?" Most people are satisfied with the mere title they receive in reply: "I'm a _____ (fill in the blank)." Furthermore, most people have a basic concept of many trades or professions, such as plumber, doctor, electrician, nurse, policeman, and so forth. However, when I am asked what I do for a living, I always receive a polite yet uncertain smile, a slight nod of the head, and, following a short pause, the inevitable follow-up question: "What does an occupational therapist do?"

The answers that I used to give were usually long, disjointed, complicated, and, yes, boring. To remedy this, I spent many years editing, splicing, revising, and polishing my definition of the profession until it became what would be called in the news business a "sound bite." I will share my personal, party-version definition with you later in this chapter. First, let's look at how occupational therapy is officially defined.

In 2004, the American Occupational Therapy Association (AOTA) began to revise its official definition of the profession:

> *Occupational therapy is the use of purposeful activity (unique feature) or interventions to promote health and achieve functional outcomes (generic goals of most health care fields). Achieving functional outcomes means to develop, improve, or restore the highest possible level of independence (purpose/goal) of any individual who is limited by a physical injury or illness, a dysfunctional condition, a cognitive impairment, a psychosocial dysfunction, a mental illness, a developmental or learning disability, or an adverse environmental condition (population served). Assessment means the use of skilled observation or evaluation by the administration and interpretation of standardized or non-standardized tests and measurements to identify areas for occupational therapy services.*
>
> *Occupational therapy services include, but are not limited to:*
>
> 1. *the assessment, treatment, and education of or consultation with the individual, family, or other persons (process); or*
> 2. *interventions directed toward developing, improving, or restoring daily living skills, work readiness or work performance, play skills or leisure capacities, or enhancing educational performance skills (objectives); or*

3. *providing for the development, improvement, or restoration of sensorimotor, oral-motor, perceptual, or neuromuscular functioning; or emotional, motivational, cognitive, or psychosocial components of performance (objectives).*

These services may require assessment of the need for and use of interventions such as the design, development, adaptation, application, or training in the use of assistive technology devices; the design, fabrication, or application of rehabilitation technology such as selected orthotic devices; training in the use of assistive technology, orthotic, or prosthetic devices; the application of physical agent modalities as an adjunct to or in preparation for purposeful activity; the use of ergonomic principles; the adaptation of environments and processes to enhance functional performance; or the promotion of health and wellness (means).

Whew! Okay, take a short break before you continue. No wonder no one talked to me at parties. I believe that if you cannot get your point across to people in 10 seconds or less, you have lost them completely. I realized that if I wanted to educate people about the profession of occupational therapy, I would need to immediately grab their attention and leave them wanting to know more.

Webster's New Collegiate Dictionary (1973) defines *occupation* as "an activity in which one engages" and "the principal business of one's life" (p. 794). It then defines *therapy* as "a remedial treatment of a bodily disorder . . . designed or serving to bring about social adjustment" (p. 1210). There you have it. By combining these two simple definitions, you have the basis of a profession that has been around for over 80 years. Occupational therapy uses purposeful activities, or occupations, to engage the patient in the therapeutic process in order to treat a physical, developmental (that is, occurring at birth or during childhood), or psychosocial disability, thus allowing that person to function in and contribute to society within the confines of his disability. To use my personal party definition, occupational therapy helps people to do the things that are most important to them (14 words!). What we do is not complicated at all; how we accomplish our goals is what gets complicated.

So, what is the big mystery about occupational therapy? Why is it so hard for practitioners to define and for the general public to understand? The major problem occurs in the sub-definitions of what comprises "occupation"; most people think of paid employment when they hear the term. I cannot count the number of patients who have said to me, "I've worked all of my life and now I'm retired. Why do you want to teach me a new occupation?" We all engage in occupations from the moment we are born until, hopefully, the day we die. Occupation is what truly separates human beings from other species upon our planet. It is not the fact that we have an opposable thumb—so do apes. It is not that we manufacture and use tools—so do apes. What truly sets us apart from all other species is the fact that we, as human beings, engage in deliberate, purposeful activities and occupations. These occupations can be for survival, such as food gathering (grocery shopping), or they can be for fun, such as playing a game of tennis. Occupations can even be inane time-fillers or pastimes, such as building a house of cards.

Another important factor that separates human beings from other creatures is our ability to recognize time and use it effectively to our advantage. John Shelby Spong (2005) has described humans as "living in a medium called time that has a past that can be remembered and a future that can be anticipated" (p. 285). Adolf Meyer (1922), who was very aware of the importance of time to people, observed that people organize time in terms of doing things, or, occupation.

The Importance of Occupation

Regardless of what we do for occupation, its primary purpose is to help us to grow as human beings or, at the very least, to prevent us from stagnating, decompensating, and ultimately dying. Without occupation, there is no growth. Without growth, there is only stagnation and death.

Indeed, death can, and often does, occur long before an individual exhales for the last time. Boredom is a form of "living death." A person with "too much time on his hands" may engage in mischief or criminal behavior. Thus, the expression "idle hands are the devil's playground." I refer to these behaviors as *dys-occupation* or *mal-occupation*. People who are continually bored will often spiral into depression, substance abuse, and all of the problems associated with these disorders. Noted psychiatrist Thomas Szasz has said that "Boredom is the feeling that everything is a waste of time; serenity that nothing is" (http://www.quoteworld.org). French military commander Le Duc de Levis (1720–1787) likewise noted that "Boredom is a sickness, the cure for which is work (occupation)" (http://www.quoteworld.org).

At the other end of the spectrum is the feeling that one has too much to do and that there is not enough time to finish what needs to be done; therefore, the challenge of the activity is too great. This feeling leads to anxiety and, in many people, a feeling of being overwhelmed and unable to complete or even participate in a task. Consequently, nothing gets done.

When one is able to reach a point in an activity where the activity is interesting enough to keep one's attention (eliminating boredom) and easy enough to prevent anxiety and frustration, one has achieved the state of function known as "flow." When one reaches the state of flow, one becomes lost in concentration and frequently loses track of time. Many people in the state of flow lose the perception of pain; that is, they become so engrossed in what they are doing that they no longer feel any pain that may have been previously bothering them.

Imagine yourself—a healthy, active individual—involved in a serious accident that leaves you unable to perform the simplest activities, such as feeding yourself, brushing your hair, or getting dressed. You lie in bed, day after day, watching the monotonous parade of television shows, occasionally asking someone to change the channel. How would you feel? Would you be energized? Happy? Fulfilled? Or would you be angry, depressed, and contemplating suicide?

You would be beyond miserable. You would be unable to help yourself or support your family. You would be unable to contribute to society and, instead, you would be a drain on others' resources. All of us have a need to contribute to society in some way, however small. Some people need to be involved in local, state, or national government. Some contribute through music and the arts. Some do what they can to make the world a better place. Some just want to get through the workday, pay their taxes, and raise their families in the best way they know how. To be unable to act independently on a daily basis and to contribute to society is unthinkable to the vast majority of people—and yet, there are tens of thousands who are in that position at any given time.

Each of us is only an accident away from a disability. This could happen to you. In fact, this scenario occurs throughout the world on a daily basis: there are car accidents, wars, diseases, and mental breakdowns. All of these terrible occurrences have one thing in common—they impair an individual's ability to participate in her occupation of choice.

The Multiple Roles of the Occupational Therapist

It is the job and, more importantly, the duty of the occupational therapist to assist these individuals to achieve their maximal abilities in their preferred occupations. To meet this noble goal, it is necessary to assist

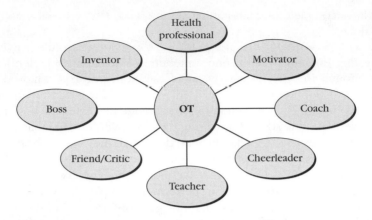

Figure 1-1. The many roles of the OT

the individual in sorting out what it is that she would like to achieve, and to provide the individual with the skills and encouragement needed to master the environment and reach full potential. To this end, the occupational therapist takes on a variety of roles: teacher, coach, inventor, friend, boss, cheerleader, motivator, critic, and health care professional (see Figure 1–1).

Teacher

Teaching is an integral part of occupational therapy. We frequently must teach a person something that is entirely new to him, or sometimes we must teach him how to do something that he could do at one time, but no longer can. Sometimes it is necessary to teach people how to do something in a new and different way.

For example, John was completely independent in all aspects of his life. One day, however, he had a stroke that left him unable to use his dominant right arm and hand. John became frustrated and depressed because he could no longer perform the simplest tasks, such as getting dressed, buttoning his clothes, or opening containers. Through the educational process of occupational therapy, he was able to relearn how to perform these tasks using different approaches and is now able to continue to live an independent lifestyle.

Coach

A coach is one who trains another by instruction, demonstration, and practice (Webster's New Collegiate Dictionary). Although most of us think of coaching as an athletic occupation, we find coaches in many areas of life; this is especially true of occupational therapy. Coaching is an extension of teaching. The occupational therapist must first teach the activity, then demonstrate it, and, finally, allow the patient to practice it in order to incorporate it into his own habit patterns. This is similar to how medical students learn to perform surgery, known as the "see one, do one, teach one" approach.

Inventor

An individual's environment must frequently be adapted in order to help her interact effectively with the environment to perform a given activity or task. This is where the inventor—or "MacGyver"—comes in. An occupational therapist once said, "Necessity is the mother of invention" (okay, okay, so it was really Plato). Nevertheless, nowhere is this statement truer than in occupational therapy.

To me, this is the most exciting and, often, the most challenging aspect of the profession. Every person is a unique individual, and every individual's problems are therefore unique. Inventing or fabricating a device that allows someone to participate in a desired activity can be a truly wonderful feeling for both the therapist and the patient. These devices can be as simple and "low tech" as building a spoon to allow someone with weak or arthritic hands to feed himself, obtaining a commercially available reaching device to allow someone who cannot bend over to reach items located on the floor, or utilizing high-tech additions such as infrared control switches to allow a child with cerebral palsy to independently operate a favorite toy or a computer.

Friend

Friends help friends; "That's what friends do," said Donkey to Shrek in the 2001 film *Shrek*. As a therapist, it is beneficial to the therapeutic relationship to be friends with your patients. You need to listen to them and hear their concerns; share their joys and sorrows; laugh with them and sometimes cry with them. All of these things are what friends do. They will also facilitate the therapeutic process and assist in motivating the patient.

It is just as important, however, to know where the invisible line between professional and personal involvement is situated in a relationship. Health care professionals too often become unduly involved with a patient or family because they not only step over the line, they never even saw it to begin with. The professional relationship must be maintained at all times during the active treatment process. To not do so can result in unrealistic expectations, a failed therapeutic relationship, and, ultimately, professional burnout.

This is not to say that you cannot establish a friendship with your patients; however, a nonprofessional relationship should not begin until after the therapeutic relationship is officially over.

Motivator

Friends often face a problem when another friend does not want to do something that needs to be done for her own good. As uncomfortable as it may be, sometimes you have to be a boss and force—I mean, strongly encourage—your patient to participate. This, of course, must be done in a friendly, loving, professional manner. If you are too pushy, you may get no cooperation at all; a fine line, indeed.

Akin to the boss is the cheerleader. Encouraging the individual in a positive manner is sometimes necessary and usually effective in getting someone to participate in activities. Using cheers such as "I *know* you can do it!" gives the patient the little push that he might need.

You must be a motivator to encourage your patients to do the best that they can, whether that means being a boss or a cheerleader. Both of these techniques are *external motivators*, which come from outside of the individual. External motivation can be positive, in the form of rewards and compensation, or it can be negative, in the form of threats or punishment. The best form of motivation comes from *internal motivators*, which reside inside the individual and cause them to do things because they want to do them or because it makes them feel good inside. Internal motivation is a push that, physiologically, produces endorphins—the body's natural painkillers.

In my own professional experience in hospice, I have seen internal motivators allow terminally ill individuals to live far beyond their prognoses because they had something to live for and were able to continue to participate in life. My mentor and best friend, the late Kent Nelson Tigges, MS, OTR (1983), said that occupational therapy provided the terminally ill "a hope without a future: a future without time" (personal communication, 1983). This is only made possible by providing the individual with the tools needed to find her personal intrinsic motivation. As the old saying goes, "You can lead a horse to water, but you can't make him drink." So it is with people. People must *want* to do something if they expect to get any enjoyment out of it. Another great occupational therapist once said, "Enthusiasm is the mother of effort and without it nothing great was ever achieved" (alright, it was really Ralph Waldo Emerson).

Critic

It is sometimes necessary to be a critic. When I say this, I do not mean that you should point out your patient's flaws and shortcomings. A critic is one who analyzes, evaluates, and expresses reasoned opinions about a patient's performance. In essence, to criticize is to provide feedback. This feedback must be provided in a positive manner; people learn through *constructive* criticism. No one likes negative criticism and most people ignore it, rebel against it, or throw in the towel and give up. We cannot afford to have our patients rebel or give up during the therapeutic process. We must help them to succeed in reaching their therapy goals.

Consummate Professional

Finally, an occupational therapist is, above all, a health professional. The occupational therapist and occupational therapy assistant are members of the health care team—all of whom have a part to play in the patient's recovery. The required scientific education to become an occupational therapist or an occupational therapy assistant includes anatomy, the study of the structure of the human body, physiology, the study of the function of the human body; kinesiology, the study of movement; neuroanatomy, the study of the structure of the nervous system; neuroscience, the study of the function of the nervous system; sociology, the study of group behavior in society; and psychology, the study of the functions of the mind and behavior.

Many occupational therapists like to point out that occupational therapy is a "holistic" profession and that other professions are "reductionistic," thus implying that occupational therapy is better than the rest. The holistic rubric stems from the fact that occupational therapy considers both the body *and* the mind rather than one or the other, as is so often typical of many other health professions. Holistic does *not* mean that occupational therapy must attend to *all* aspects of the patient's recovery; that is not possible within the scope of the practice. Occupational therapy addresses the patients' occupational needs and those things that hinder occupational role performance. This is more than enough to address.

Flexibility in Practice

An occupational therapist or occupational therapy assistant must always be flexible. As we all know, nothing in life is perfect, and, frequently, things do not go as planned. For example, we may spend weeks planning a special picnic and, when the day finally arrives, it snows. The inflexible person shouts and swears and pouts. The flexible person sets up the picnic on the garage floor and has a good time despite the inclement weather. The same can happen in therapy; although a given activity has been meticulously planned, something untoward may occur that throws a monkey wrench into the process.

Presume, for example, that a therapist develops a brilliant new set-up to help a client increase his upper extremity strength. The therapist goes to the patient's room to bring him to his scheduled therapy session, only to find that the client has just soiled himself. The inflexible therapist might say, "Well, I guess we'll just have to wait until tomorrow for therapy; by the time you are cleaned up, it will be too late for therapy today." The flexible therapist, on the other hand, would say, "Well, we can wait until tomorrow for the strengthening program. Why don't we take this opportunity to work on your dressing and bathing skills?" The flexible scenario is a win-win proposition for everyone.

A relevant story exists about Mahatma Gandhi, the Indian statesman who helped India gain its independence from Great Britain through peaceful means. Gandhi was always sought out by others for his sage advice. One day, a woman who had been waiting for over 10 hours in the hot sun to see him asked him to tell her daughter not to eat sweets. Gandhi looked at the little girl and then looked up at her mother. "I cannot tell her that today," he said. "Come back in one month." The mother, visibly upset, agreed and set off to her home in the next village. One month later, she returned and waited another 10 hours to see him. This time, when she approached him with the same request, he looked the little girl in the eyes and said, "Do not eat sweets, little one." Her exasperated mother looked at Gandhi and asked, "Why didn't you just tell her that last month?" He looked at the frustrated woman and calmly replied, "Because, madam, last month I was eating sweets myself."

A Sense of Humor Goes a Long Way

An important part of being a professional is possessing a sense of humor. For the occupational therapist, as with any health care professional, a sense of humor is not just helpful, it is essential. A well-developed sense of humor can help the therapist to put the client at ease and, therefore, contribute to the successful therapeutic relationship. President Dwight D. Eisenhower (1890–1969) once stated, "A sense of humor is part of the art of leadership, of getting along with people, of getting things done." A sense of humor in occupational therapy does not necessarily imply the telling of jokes or resorting to slapstick behavior, but it does include the ability to laugh at oneself and to see the humor in a situation, even if that situation appears to be dire.

The best type of humor to use, in my opinion, is the self-deprecating kind (I used to jokingly say "self-defecating" humor, but many people mistook my intentional malapropism as a sign of stupidity). Self-deprecating humor is that type of humor where one makes fun of oneself rather than someone else. It is easy to kid and mock others, but this is also a sure way to distance others from you. By mocking oneself, you can show others that you are a self-confident individual. Max Eastman (1883–1969), a noted author and journalist, once said, "It is the ability to take a joke, not make one, that proves you have a sense of humor."

Perhaps the most important aspect of a sense of humor is its ability to keep you focused, refreshed, and to prevent psychological burnout—a condition caused by unrelieved stress and marked by feelings of powerlessness, hopelessness, frustration, interpersonal detachment, and general dissatisfaction. Burnout is real and very common; if untreated, it can develop into clinical depression.

The people who are most affected by burnout are those who work with other people, including health care professionals. A sense of humor can contribute to one's mental well-being and help to stave off the detrimental effects of stress and burnout. If you were to drive your car day in and day out, without ever changing the oil or lubricating the chassis, eventually your car would wear out and cease to function. Think of your sense of humor as the lubrication that allows you to function at an optimal level each day; check your oil level frequently!

SUMMARY

Occupational therapy is a vital, yet often misunderstood, health care profession. The occupational therapists use activities that are important to the patient in order to meet therapeutic goals. Although what the OT does is fairly straightforward, the methods to achieve goals are varied, and sometimes it is difficult to see how things fit into the big picture.

The occupational therapist must wear a number of professional hats in order to facilitate the therapeutic process and stir internal motivation within the patient. These hats include: teacher, coach, inventor, friend, boss, cheerleader, motivator, critic, and consummate professional. A sense of humor is vital to facilitate the therapeutic relationship and prevent burnout in the therapist.

References

Merriam-Webster's new collegiate dictionary (3rd ed.). (1973). Springfield, MA: Merriam-Webster.

Meyer, A. (1922). The philosophy of occupational therapy. *Archives of Occupational Therapy, 1*(1), 5.

Mosby's medical, nursing, and allied health dictionary (5th ed.). (1998). St. Louis, MO: Mosby.

Quote World Web site. (n.d.). Retrieved 12/02/05 from http://www.quoteworld.org

Spong, J. S. (2005). *The sins of scripture.* New York, NY: HarperCollins.

Tigges, K. N. (1983). Occupational therapy in hospice. In C. A. Corr & D. M. Corr (Eds.), *Hospice care: principles and practice.* New York, NY: Springer Publishing Company.

CHAPTER 2

A Brief History of Occupational Therapy

Chapter Goals

At the conclusion of this chapter, the reader should:

- Have a basic understanding of the early days of medicine and psychiatry
- Have a basic understanding of the moral treatment movement.
- Understand the roots of the profession of occupational therapy.
- Have a basic knowledge of the birth and growth of the profession from 1918 until the present day.

INTRODUCTION

No book on occupational therapy would be complete without the requisite chapter on the history of the profession; this book is no different. As the profession of occupational therapy is not all that old, this chapter isn't too long. In fact, I have tried to condense the early history a bit and focus on the more relevant recent history of the profession.

This chapter will give a brief history of modern medicine and psychiatry, warts and all. It also describes the moral treatment movement of the 19th century, which set the tone for the origin of occupational therapy.

A Brief Prelude to Modern Medicine

Occupation has always been an integral part of human civilization. One of the earliest written accounts of occupation can be found in the Bible (Genesis 2:15): "The Lord God took the man and put him in the Garden of Eden to work it and take care of it." The philosopher Plato (427 BCE–347 BCE) advised, "Apply yourself . . . without effort you cannot be prosperous. Though the land be good, you cannot have an abundant crop without cultivation." Our ancestors participated in occupations such as hunting and gathering, farming, and manufacturing, as well as play. By extension, one could argue that there has always been occupational therapy.

Disease has also been an integral part of human civilization, though the ways in which it has been addressed have changed over the years. In biblical accounts, people with leprosy (now known as Hansen's disease) were ostracized or rejected by society at large and forced to fend for themselves by begging, or they were herded into leper colonies far removed from the general population. The blind and disabled were also forced to rely on the generosity of others. There were no systems in place to help those who could not help themselves or who were unable to contribute to society.

Those unlucky enough to be mentally ill had even bigger problems. Mental illness was typically associated with demonic possession or witchcraft, and the treatments available for these afflictions were, shall we say, not desirable. Examination of prehistoric human skeletons have shown that many of these individuals were the unfortunate recipients of a surgical— or, in some respects, religious—procedure known as **trephining.** This involved boring a hole in the skull, probably with a sharp rock (ouch!), in order to release demons or evil spirits. If the poor souls survived this procedure, which was most certainly performed without anesthesia, they probably walked around with open holes in their skulls until they died from inevitable infection. This, of course, led to the adage "I need that like I need a hole in my head!"

Persons suffering from depression and other disorders of the mind in ancient Greece were often accompanied to the top of a high cliff and thrown into the sea, far below. The idea was to shock them out of their disorder and heal them. There was just that one unfortunate side effect: death due to massive trauma or drowning.

Those who were fortunate enough to survive these cures, however, had nowhere to turn for help and no way to support themselves. Many of these individuals ended up in mental institutions or, more often than not, in prisons. In fairness to the Greeks, it should be noted that Hippocrates, the "Father of Medicine," did attempt to address disease— both physical and psychological—from an objective standpoint and, to a certain extent, managed to remove some of the stigma and supernatural references.

In the Middle Ages, however, the supernatural references to disease were reprised, and mental illness, in particular, was believed to be caused by demonic possession and witchcraft. Treatments had improved somewhat since the days of trephining and throwing people off of cliffs; now people were exorcized using such methods as torture, drowning, and burning at the stake. This, of course, was done with the victim's best interests in mind, for no one really wanted to serve as a vessel for the devil; and so, it is assumed, most of these individuals gladly participated in the healing and cleansing rituals.

The Rise and Fall of the Moral Treatment Movement

Most occupational therapy scholars agree that the seeds of the profession were sown in the 18th century, during the Age of Enlightenment, which is referred to by some as the Age of Reason. Two individuals, in particular, set the stage for the profession of occupational therapy: Philippe Pinel and William Tuke.

Philippe Pinel (1745–1826) was a French physician best known for his *traitement moral* of the mentally ill. At his insistence, thousands of mentally ill patients were released from their chains, and treatments such as **bloodletting, purging,** and **blistering** were eliminated and replaced with more humane methods, including physical exercise, purposeful work, or ergotherapy (Greek for "work"), the precursor to occupational therapy (see Figure 2–1). Dr. Pinel was also present at the guillotine execution of King Louise XVI—talk about bloodletting and purging!

William Tuke (1732–1822) was a Quaker businessman and philanthropist who was outraged by the inhumane treatment of inmates at the York Asylum in England. His efforts at reform resulted in the opening, in 1796, of the York Retreat for the Humane Care of the Insane. Much like his French contemporary, Pinel, Tuke's methods included the removal of chains and the therapeutic use of occupation in the treatment of the

The practice of "therapeutic" bloodletting has been around since the times of ancient Egyptian dynasties and was commonly practiced well into the 19th century. People believed that many physical and psychological disorders could be alleviated simply by the drawing off of blood.

For centuries, it was believed that illness was caused by an imbalance of one or more of the four humors contained in the body: yellow bile, black bile, blood, and phlegm. When the four humors were in balance, the individual was healthy and "in good humor." Bloodletting was a way to restore this balance.

In addition to cutting hair, barbers would often bleed people. They would hang blood-soaked white bandages outside of their establishments as a way of advertising this aspect of their business; this served as the original form of the modern red and white (and sometimes blue) striped barber pole.

George Washington developed a throat infection in 1799 that, today, would be treated with antibiotics. His physicians, however, used bloodletting as a means to cure his ailment. Unfortunately, they took so much of his blood over the course of a few days that our first president died.

Believe it or not, bloodletting is still practiced today for certain conditions. As with so many questionable practices, the name has been changed: bloodletting is now called phlebotomy and is used on patients with certain blood conditions, such as *hemochromatosis,* a condition in which too much iron exists in the blood. To relieve this condition, blood is removed until the patient is rendered mildly anemic; the removed blood is frequently used in transfusions.

Figure 2-1. Some Fun Facts about Bloodletting

mentally ill. This approach was in stark contrast to many of Tuke's peers, who advocated "noninjurious torture," which included being chained naked in cold, dank cells, starved, beaten, and exhibited to paying visitors. One of the best known of these facilities was Bethlehem Hospital in London, better known as Bedlam (Rosen, Fox, & Gregory, 1972).

The **moral treatment** movement continued to gather followers into the 19th century, bolstered by the works of Benjamin Rush and Dorothea Dix.

Benjamin Rush, known as the "Father of American Psychiatry," led a campaign to improve the lot of mentally ill patients in the United States. A true Renaissance man, Rush was an advocate of women's rights, the abolition of slavery, and the improvement of hospital conditions. Additionally, he was one of the signers of the Declaration of Independence. Talk about a busy guy!

Although he was censured for his advocacy of bloodletting, he did a great deal to improve the understanding of the mentally ill and to improve the conditions in which they lived. Shortly before his death in 1813, he published *Medical Inquiries and Observations upon the Diseases of the Mind,* the first psychiatric textbook in the United States.

Despite Rush's work, conditions for the mentally ill were slow to change. In 1841, Dorothea Lynde Dix, a social reformer, was appalled at the treatment of the mentally ill in Massachusetts. She discovered that many of the prisoners in local jails had not committed any crimes but were, in fact, mentally ill. She soon realized that the mentally ill were poorly treated, regardless of their lodgings—be it at home, in prison, or in a poorhouse.

Dix, the daughter of an alcoholic, abusive father, worked tirelessly to improve the lot of the mentally ill, not just in her home state of Massachusetts but in other states, as well. As a result of her efforts, the number of mental health hospitals in the United States increased tenfold. Dix herself played a direct role in founding 32 of these new facilities.

Sadly, and despite Dix's noble efforts, the moral treatment movement began to decline in the years following the Civil War. The reasons for this decline were many: the social and economic strain placed on the recently reunited country, the increase in the number of poor immigrants, racial discrimination, and lack of legislation, to name a few. No one had been mentored to carry on Dix's work following her pauper's death in 1887. Thus, the treatment of the mentally ill began its steady decline into premoral treatment levels (see Figure 2–2).

The Early 20th Century and the Birth of Occupational Therapy

Following the turn of the 20th century, a number of individuals began to employ the concept of occupation as a means of therapeutic modality. The lives of these individuals eventually crossed, and, ultimately, the profession of occupational therapy was born.

Adolf Meyer, a Swiss-American physician, began to reevaluate how psychiatrists were treating patients. He disagreed with the prevailing reductionistic view of the patient into organs and systems, and preferred to view the patient from a holistic perspective—including the understanding of the patient from a biographical, educational, familial, and artistic perspective; this perspective was coined *psychobiology.* His work with psychiatric patients, from the very start, included the use of occupation.

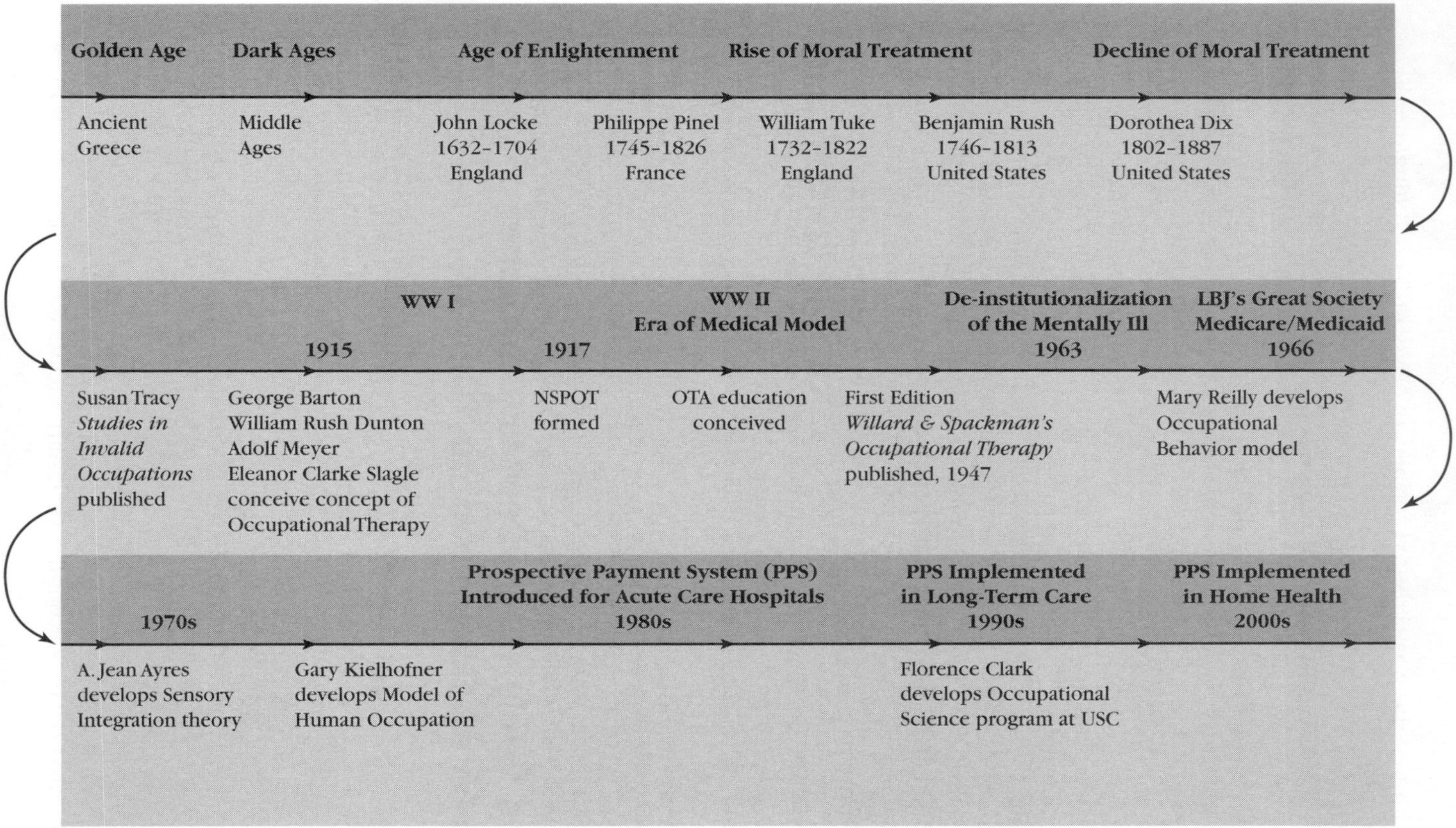

Golden Age — Dark Ages — Age of Enlightenment — Rise of Moral Treatment — Decline of Moral Treatment

- Ancient Greece
- Middle Ages
- John Locke, 1632–1704, England
- Philippe Pinel, 1745–1826, France
- William Tuke, 1732–1822, England
- Benjamin Rush, 1746–1813, United States
- Dorothea Dix, 1802–1887, United States

WW I — Age of Enlightenment — Rise of Moral Treatment — WW II / Era of Medical Model — De-institutionalization of the Mentally Ill, 1963 — LBJ's Great Society Medicare/Medicaid, 1966

- Susan Tracy, *Studies in Invalid Occupations* published
- 1915
- George Barton, William Rush Dunton, Adolf Meyer, Eleanor Clarke Slagle conceive concept of Occupational Therapy
- 1917 — NSPOT formed
- OTA education conceived
- First Edition *Willard & Spackman's Occupational Therapy* published, 1947
- Mary Reilly develops Occupational Behavior model

Prospective Payment System (PPS) Introduced for Acute Care Hospitals, 1980s — PPS Implemented in Long-Term Care, 1990s — PPS Implemented in Home Health, 2000s

- A. Jean Ayres develops Sensory Integration theory
- 1970s — Gary Kielhofner develops Model of Human Occupation
- Florence Clark develops Occupational Science program at USC

Figure 2-2. Occupational Therapy Historical Timeline

He emphasized a balance in peoples' lives between self-care, work, play/leisure, rest, and sleep. His thoughts and writings eventually formed the bedrock upon which the philosophy of occupational therapy was built. Based on his work, Meyer came to be known as the "Dean of American Psychiatry" ("Father of American Psychiatry" was already taken by Benjamin Rush, you may recall).

In the early years of the 20th century, a nurse by the name of Susan E. Tracy began to use activities and occupations with her patients. She noticed early on that patients who were occupied with an activity were more pleasant than those who languished in bed. Tracy encouraged the performance of activities and stressed the importance of a beautiful finished product. Tracy and her students came to be known as "occupational nurses." Although not an occupational therapist herself, Tracy certainly laid the groundwork for the development of the profession. In 1913, she authored what might be considered the first occupational therapy text, *Studies in Invalid Occupation: A Manual for Nurses and Attendants.*

Another important figure in the establishment of occupational therapy was George Edward Barton. Barton (no relation to Clara Barton, the founder of the Red Cross) was an architect who contracted tuberculosis and ultimately became involved in the quest for better services for hospital patients. He saw the need for hospital patients not only to recover from their illnesses, but also to return home and to work. To this end, he established Consolation House—a precursor to the modern rehabilitation hospital—in Clifton Springs, New York, near Rochester, where patients not only received medical treatment for their afflictions, but attention was paid to their social history, education, and training, as well. Clifton Springs is thus considered the birthplace of occupational therapy.

Another prominent founder, and perhaps the most prolific, was William Rush Dunton (not to be confused with Benjamin Rush). Dunton was a physician who worked with psychiatric patients for most of his career. He, too, saw the great benefits that occupation had upon his patients. He regularly encouraged his patients to participate in occupations when they were ready to do so; these activities were graded so as not to exhaust the patient. Unlike Susan Tracy, Dunton felt that the end result of the activity was not nearly as important as the actual performance of the activity itself.

Finally, Eleanor Clarke Slagle (nee Ela Clark), a social work student, can be considered the first occupational therapist. She utilized occupation with her patients and implemented a technique of Adolf Meyers', known as **habit training,** among long-term psychiatric patients to help them enjoy a semblance of temporal stability. Slagle established the first professional school for occupational therapists in Chicago and eventually became the first female president of the American Occupational Therapy Association (AOTA), in 1919.

Inevitably, the paths of these individuals crossed, and, in 1917, the National Society for the Promotion of Occupational Therapy (NSPOT) was formed and incorporated, with George Barton as its first president. In 1923, NSPOT changed its name to the American Occupational Therapy Association (AOTA), which it remains to this day.

Baptism by Fire: The War Years, 1917–1945

The new profession of occupational therapy could not have come about at a more opportune time in American history. With the United States' entry into the "Great War" (now known as World War I) came an influx of wounded soldiers needing therapy. In addition to those with serious physical injuries and amputations, there were a great number of soldiers with psychological wounds—most notably, **shell shock** (now known as post-traumatic stress disorder, or PTSD). These soldiers filled the hospitals and were tended to by reconstruction aides (later known as occupational therapists) who provided them with occupational activities to help mend their minds and bodies.

The medical emergency that resulted from World War I officially ended in 1921, and occupational therapy began to take its place in the world of medicine. Because occupational therapy views the patient as a person first and a diagnosis second (Tigges & Marcil, 1988), the psychological, physical, and social aspects of the patient's life were weighed with equal consideration.

True to its roots in the moral treatment movement, many occupational therapy programs were ensconced in psychiatric hospitals. The crafts used by both therapists and patients, particularly basketry, came to symbolize life in a mental hospital. Thus, the derisive term "basket weaver" came to refer to those institutionalized for mental illness.

The profession began to expand and rationalize its existence throughout the 1920s, 30s, and 40s. In 1947, the first edition of *Willard and Spackman's Occupational Therapy*—the "bible" of occupational therapy—was published. More schools opened, and greater numbers of young women entered the field (more on the gender issue later).

The entry of the United States into World War II in 1941 brought with it a new generation of casualties. Shell shock was still a problem, only it was now known as **battle fatigue;** though the name was new, the "thousand-yard stare" remained the same. New psychiatric "cures" abounded:

prefrontal lobotomies, electroconvulsive therapy, ice baths, and insulin shock chief among them. Psychoactive drugs also made it easier to work with many patients.

Due to a wartime shortage of occupational therapists, a two-year degree program standard was drafted. Although the entry-level, four-year degree was resumed following the war's end, this set the stage for the eventual emergence of the technical-level occupational therapy assistant in the late 1950s and early 1960s.

Occupational therapists often worked during this period with those afflicted by **polio,** a contagious and highly feared neuromuscular disease infecting and disabling millions of Americans. Many of these individuals were disabled by the wasting and weakening of their skeletal muscles, leaving them unable to walk or care for themselves. Many others relied on iron lungs, large mechanical tanks that helped the patient breathe; the patient had to remain in this device at all times in order to remain alive. The boredom of this existence proved absolutely unbearable for some, and occupational therapists frequently provided diversion from this monotonous existence. These monstrous contraptions would eventually be replaced by the smaller and more efficient ventilator of modern times, which allows individuals greater mobility.

Breaking Away from the Medical Model

The 1960s was a decade of discord, revolution, and exploration in the United States; the same can be said of the occupational therapy profession. Academics and scholars within the profession were assembling new theories and **paradigms** to promote the legitimacy and impact of their work. The days of occupational therapists working only in mental hospitals were coming to an end. Men were beginning to become involved in the previously female-dominated profession in small but significant numbers, and the number of practice arenas was growing as well.

In the early 1960s, President John F. Kennedy signed into law a bill that would **deinstitutionalize** the mentally ill; that is, it released them from psychiatric hospitals and into the community. Prior to this, mentally ill patients could be, and were, held in mental hospitals for years or even decades. These individuals were now integrated into society and needed to support themselves. They needed to relearn the basic activities of daily living and social skills; these were areas where occupational therapy could be of great service.

President Lyndon B. Johnson's **Great Society** brought a number of social changes to America in the mid-1960s, including **Medicare** and

Medicaid, designed to allow everyone to benefit from improved health care. With the U.S. government now the biggest provider of health care, new vistas were opening for the occupational therapy practitioner.

Many occupational therapists began to specialize in specific areas of treatment. Many also began working with children and incorporated new techniques devised by other occupational therapists, including **sensory integration** and **neurodevelopmental training** (NDT). Others focused on spinal cord injuries and hand rehabilitation. The areas of practice, it seemed, were endless. Wherever someone was having difficulty performing occupational roles, an occupational therapist could be found (see Figure 2–3).

Another significant landmark in the history of the profession was the establishment of the first formal educational program for **certified occupational therapy assistants** (COTAs) in 1961. COTAs were trained in occupational therapy techniques, in formal one- or two-year programs, to assist occupational therapists, registered (OTRs) and to help fill the shortage of occupational therapy personnel.

Occupational therapy continued to enter into new fields of practice throughout the 1970s, 80s, and 90s, including schools, homeless shelters, prisons, hospices, home health, and private practice. Work hardening programs are designed to return workers to their jobs following a work-related injury or disability.

In the early 1980s, the federal government began a campaign to reform the Medicare system, which many felt had gotten out of control and was rife with fraud and abuse. This brought about the advent of the **prospective payment system** (PPS) to reign in the cost of Medicare, and it had a major impact on the way health care was delivered. Beginning in acute-care hospitals, patients were assigned a specific **length of stay** (LOS) depending upon their diagnosis, which was assigned to a **diagnostic related group** (DRG). In order to save money and survive financially, hospitals were forced to discharge patients as soon as possible. Thus, many patients were discharged "sooner and sicker," which resulted in readmission to the hospital and, coincidentally, the explosive growth of the home health care industry.

In the late 1990s, the PPS began to affect long-term care facilities (i.e., nursing homes). This new phase had a drastic impact upon occupational therapy personnel, as well as other health care professions. Just a few years earlier, occupational therapy had been listed among the top 10 fastest-growing professions, and hopefuls were flocking to occupational therapy educational programs; there was a corresponding growth of educational programs to meet the demand. Now, however, the unimaginable was happening: occupational therapists were actually being laid off!

Jean Ayres: Developmental occupational therapist who developed the sensory integration framework.

Florence Clark: Developed Occupational Science program at University of Southern California (USC).

Gail S. Fidler: Author of the first textbook on psychiatric occupational therapy in 1954.

Gary Kielhofner: Developed the Model of Human Occupation (MOHO).

Lela J. Llorens: Renowned for her work with children with mental health problems, and developmental theory and adaptation over the life span. Dr. Llorens is one of the first African-Americans of prominence within the profession.

Anne Cronin Mosey: Developed Frames of Reference for psychiatric occupational therapy and the biopsychosocial model of care.

Kenneth Ottenbacher: Noted researcher in occupational therapy. Established the *Occupational Therapy Journal of Research*.

Mary Reilly: Developed Occupational Behavior model, a precursor to MOHO and occupational science.

Eleanor Clarke Slagle: The "first" occupational therapist and first female president of the American Occupational Therapy Association (AOTA), she expanded the concept of habit training. The Eleanor Clarke Slagle Lecture is named for her.

Clare S. Spackman: Coauthor of *Willard and Spackman's Occupational Therapy*. She was prominent in the World Federation of Occupational Therapists (WFOT).

Wilma West: Promoted a shift away from tertiary care to one of disease prevention and health promotion. The AOTA's Wilma West Library is named for her.

Helen Willard: Coauthor of *Willard and Spackman's Occupational Therapy*. Ms. Willard was involved in occupational therapy for over 60 years as a therapist, educator, past president of the AOTA, and architect of the WFOT.

Figure 2-3. Notable People in Occupational Therapy History

If ever a dark period existed in the history of the profession, this was it. Students began to seek other professions, and enrollment in occupational therapy schools dropped precipitately. Many programs closed down due to waning enrollments.

As with most situations in life, however, the pendulum slowly swung the other way, and equilibrium was once again restored. Enrollments in

OT programs now continue to climb, and the job market is once again growing; the need for occupational therapy services is still strong. The AOTA currently has approximately 50,000 active members working in a broad spectrum of practice areas.

SUMMARY

Although the occupational therapy profession was officially established in 1917, the seeds for the profession were planted hundreds of years ago, beginning with the moral treatment movement. The human need for occupation is innate, and the use of occupation in the recovery process is extremely important to the disabled, regardless of their diagnosis. The profession has grown steadily since its inception and continues to do so into the 21st century.

References

Bing, R. K. (1981). Occupational therapy revisited: A paraphrastic journey. *American Journal of Occupational Therapy. 35*, 499–518.

Rosen, E., Gregory, I., & Fox, R. E. (1972). *Abnormal psychology* (2nd ed.). London: W. B. Saunders Company.

Sabonis-Chafee, B., & Hussey, S. M. (1998). *Introduction to occupational therapy* (2nd ed.). St. Louis, MO: Mosby.

Schwartz, K. B. (2003). The history of occupational therapy. In E. B. Crepeau, E. S. Cohn, & B. A. B. Schell (Eds.), *Willard and Spackman's occupational therapy* (10th ed., pp. 5–13). Philadelphia, PA: Lippincott Williams & Wilkins.

Tigges, K. N., & Marcil, W. M. (1988). *Terminal and life-threatening illness: An occupational behavior approach*. Thorofare, NJ: Slack, Inc.

PART II

Occupational Therapy: How It Works

TEACH A MAN TO FISH, AND YOU FEED HIM FOR A LIFETIME. UNLESS HE DOESN'T LIKE SUSHI—THEN YOU ALSO HAVE TO TEACH HIM TO COOK.
- AUREN HOFFMAN, HERALD PHILOSOPHER

CHAPTER 3

Basic Concepts of Occupational Therapy

Chapter Goals

At the conclusion of this chapter, the reader should:

- Understand the difference between the occupational roles of work, self-care, and play and leisure.
- Understand the importance of rest and sleep.
- Understand the importance of a balance of occupational roles.
- Understand the importance of time management.
- Understand the importance of applying principles to practice.

INTRODUCTION

This chapter will further define occupational therapy by covering the components of occupation: work, self-care, play and leisure, rest, and sleep. It will further explore the importance of a balance between each of these components in terms of optimal physical and mental health. Related to this balance is the concept of time management, and how individuals either use time or are used by time. Finally, this chapter will explain how occupational therapy theory and principles can be applied to realistic practice.

Defining Occupation

When I tell someone that I am an occupational therapist, that person inevitably says, "Oh, you help people to find jobs." When I say "not really," they become confused. "Well, what does occupation mean, then?"

For some, this question elicits a long, drawn-out explanation. For me, the answer is simple: an occupation is anything that someone does, on a regular basis, as part of who he is as a person. This includes dressing, bathing, eating, toileting, working at a paying job, volunteering, enjoying a hobby, raising children, or any number of other activities.

As far as occupational therapists are concerned, occupations are divided into three main categories: work, self-care, and play and leisure.

Work

Work means many things to many people. Mosey (1973) defined work as "an individual's major occupation and what a person does to make money" (p. 18). Cawood (1975) described work as all types of productive activity, paid or unpaid, regardless of the locale, while Shannon (1970) believed it to be the arena in which individuals attempt to validate themselves. Regardless of the multitude of definitions, work is essentially how people define themselves in our society. Work consumes most of our everyday lives, often to the exclusion of other activities.

When two people meet at a party or in some other social setting, one of the first questions asked is "What do you do for a living?" The other person may reply, "I'm an actress." However, she may leave unspoken the fact that she also works as a waitress to support herself, that she is a mother of two young children, and that she is responsible for cooking, cleaning, and shopping for them. All of these activities are classified as work.

We judge people based on the types of work that they do or don't do. Some occupations are presumed to be better than others, such as physician, lawyer, or teacher as opposed to automobile mechanic, farmer, or garbage collector. Every occupation has its place in society, however, and society as a whole needs each of these workers. Have you ever considered what would happen if there were no auto mechanics, farmers, or garbage collectors?

On the other hand, we may view with disdain—consciously or unconsciously—those who do not work. We often perceive the unemployed as lazy parasites who make no contribution to society, even though there may be a very good reason why they are unemployed: lack of skills or education, "downsizing" or "workforce reduction" (a couple of my favorite euphemisms), physical or mental illness, or some other misfortune. Indeed, the unemployed usually do not offer the fact that they are not working. When asked, they may state their previous position or perhaps volunteer that they are "between jobs at the moment" (yet another great euphemism).

Most of us are, however, just as bothered by the "idle rich": those who do not have to work because they have all of the money they need. Our well-justified jealousy aside, we fault them for not contributing to society by working and making something of themselves.

Self-Care

Self-care is defined as "activities or tasks done routinely to maintain the client's health and well-being, considering the environment and social factors" (Trombly, 1995, p. 352). Self-care activities are things that we all do on a daily basis, such as bathing, dressing, self-feeding, toileting, and so forth. In the occupational therapy profession, these tasks are referred to as daily living skills, activities of daily living (ADLs), and instrumental activities of daily living (IADLs) (Figure 3-1). Deloach and Greer (1981) stated that people are expected to perform routine tasks, such as dressing, feeding, and grooming, before they are considered well adapted to community life. Obviously, one must be able to perform self-care activities as a prerequisite to functioning in society.

Obtaining independent self-care is a developmental process. Newborns and infants are completely dependent in all aspects of self-care; they must be fed, changed, bathed, and dressed. Gradually a child learns

ACTIVITIES OF DAILY LIVING	INSTRUMENTAL ACTIVITIES OF DAILY LIVING
Eating	Shopping, selecting food, preparing meals
Bathing	Preparing the tub/shower, cleaning bathroom
Dressing	Purchasing clothes, washing/ironing clothes
Ambulation (walking)	Driving a car
Wheelchair mobility	Using public transportation

Figure 3-1. Activities of daily living (ADLs) versus instrumental activities of daily living (IADLs)

to feed herself, use the toilet, bathe, and dress. But for many years, these activities must be supervised by adults until the child masters them.

Children who do not develop these skills, or people who lose these skills due to an accident, advanced age, or illness, are at a distinct disadvantage as members of society. They will either require assistance with these tasks, or they will need to learn how to perform them independently.

Play and Leisure

Finally, play and leisure includes any activity engaged in for its own sake. Play is often spontaneous and should always involve fun. Play can be an activity as simple as playing solitaire or Go Fish, or it might be something as complicated as an organized baseball game.

Contrary to popular belief, however, play is not all fun and games; it has a special meaning in people's lives. Play develops in a hierarchical process (Reilly, 1974). Children play all the time, but, in the process, they are learning about many different things within a nonstructured environment. The act of playing helps children learn how to interact with, and get along with, other children (and adults). Play also teaches them rules, helps them to develop physical, emotional, and social skills, and prepares them for future occupational roles. In fact, play is the antecedent to work. It has been said that play is a child's work; play helps children explore their environment in a safe manner and at their own pace. It helps them "try on" occupational roles, such as "mommy," "daddy," "teacher," and so forth.

Play offers children a safe environment in which to practice rules, skills, and roles that can be maintained or discarded for future life situations. It allows children to develop exploratory behaviors that can ultimately help foster feelings of hope for the future and trust in the environment.

Play also allows children to develop competence behaviors or skills, again in a safe environment. Children learn how to deal effectively with their environment, in order to help develop skills and habits needed to perform future roles. Success in these ventures can lead to feelings of confidence.

Finally, play helps develop achievement behaviors, as the child's behaviors result in an impact on his environment. This is important, because it generates feelings of courage toward taking risks in the interest of winning. Recent research has found that the key to happiness is not money, love, or material things; the key to happiness is taking risks. If this is true, play is the key to happiness.

If, on the other hand, play is not allowed to occur in a safe environment—if it is overshadowed by anxiety, threats, or ridicule—exploratory behaviors will not occur, and hope and trust will not emerge. This type of environment will reduce the possibility of the child developing risk-taking behaviors later in life. Think of children growing up in ghettos who later end up in gangs, or children in war zones whose thoughts focus only on daily survival rather than on play, mastery, or risk taking.

We tend to grow removed from play as we age. As we enter the world of work, adults play less and less. We develop hobbies—we may play golf or perform other avocational activities—but we seem to lose that primeval instinct to relax and play, just for the sake of play. Occasionally we may do something spontaneous and fun, and say, "I felt like a kid again!"

Some feel that leisure is earned: unless one works, one cannot enjoy leisure activities. Benjamin Franklin recognized this when he said, "Employ thy time well if one is meant to enjoy leisure". This seems like common sense, but for those who are unable to work, leisure time makes up the majority of the day and may leave them feeling as though they are not contributing to society. However, leisure is a ready substitute for the worker role and we, as a society, need to recognize this and celebrate it whenever possible.

One of my favorite episodes of the original *Twilight Zone* television show is called "Kick the Can," and it takes place in a retirement home named Sunnyvale Rest. One of the residents realizes that the secret of youth is to act young, so he organizes a group of the elderly residents to play a game of Kick the Can, much to the chagrin of some of the other residents and staff, who think that they should act their age (that is, they should sit around in rocking chairs and play checkers all day). One night, the residents go out to play Kick the Can, magically become children, and disappear from the grounds of Sunnyvale Rest—leaving the stick-in-the-mud oldsters to live out the rest of their boring lives. Ah, the magic of play!

Rest and Sleep: The Forgotten Occupations

The secret to a healthy lifestyle is a balance between work, self-care, play, rest, and sleep. We frequently forget about the rest and sleep aspects, and many people consider them one and the same. I, however, view them as two separate but extremely important aspects of occupation.

Rest is somewhat difficult to define. We all do it, but rest means different things to different people. Webster's New Collegiate Dictionary defines rest as "a bodily state characterized by minimal function and metabolic activities; freedom from activity or labor; a state of motionlessness or inactivity" (p. 987). Resting usually takes the form of a short pause while we are doing some type of activity. When we go for a hike, we take a number of short rests to give us the energy to continue. While I'm working on this chapter, I frequently stop, stand, and stretch, or I play solitaire on my computer for a while. Then I go back to what I was doing, usually with a renewed vitality (unfortunately, my wife usually comes into the room while I'm playing solitaire and thinks that I'm just goofing off).

Perhaps, rather than look at the word *rest*, we should instead look at the word *rest-ore*. When we restore something, we renew it; we bring it back to its original state of being or its original use. That is what we do when we rest: we renew ourselves. We return ourselves to a previous state that allows us to continue to participate in a given activity.

Rest appears to be turning into a thing of the past. As modern workers, we are only required by law to work 40 hours each week, which leaves us with a great deal of leisure time. However, many of us choose to work substantially longer hours each week. Even when we are not at work and are "relaxing," modern technology—such as cellular phones, wireless laptops, and BlackBerrys—allows us to stay connected 24 hours a day. Ultimately, many of us continue to work even when we're not working. What's up with that?

Rest can be a passive activity, such as sitting in a comfortable chair and listening to music, meditating, or performing progressive relaxation exercises. Rest can also be active. There are some people who are unable to rest passively and must DO SOMETHING! These individuals may consider rest to include watching television, reading, performing tai chi, yoga, or some other low-energy activity. Rest, however, is not sleep. Rest may lead to sleep, and sleep may promote rest. Nonetheless, they are two separate and distinct entities. Perhaps the best way to distinguish between rest and sleep is to think of rest as *psychological* renewal and sleep as *physical* renewal.

Sleep is a very complicated phenomenon. We all sleep, but most of us don't really know why, or what it is—and frankly, most of us don't really care. The only time we think about sleep is when we can't seem to get any (kind of like food, sex, and money). Sleep is a very active process in which our bodies may appear to be shut down, when, in fact, many invisible processes are occurring. The primary process is the alteration of brain waves, which occurs numerous times during a typical night's sleep. Essential hormones are also produced during sleep, and our tissues get a chance to rebuild.

Although sleep is important to everyone, it is particularly important to children. Studies have found that school-age children who get sufficient sleep perform better in school than those who do not. Further, children who do not get adequate amounts of sleep frequently exhibit symptoms of attention deficit disorder (ADD), which can interfere with their academic and interpersonal pursuits. Sadly, many of these children are unnecessarily put on medication, which may further impair their functioning.

On the other end of the sleep spectrum is the person who sleeps too much. Excessive sleep, or hypersomnia, is not good for most people either. Obviously, if one sleeps 12 to 15 hours a day, there isn't much time left to do anything else. The causes of excessive sleep, including clinical depression and chronic fatigue syndrome, must be determined and remedied as soon as possible.

Many things can interfere with sleep: poor scheduling, stealing time from sleep to attend to other activities (robbing Peter to pay Paul), anxiety, depression, sleep apnea, restless leg syndrome, and insomnia, to name a few. Sleep problems can have dire consequences and must be addressed quickly if people are to function adequately. Sleep is not a waste of time; it is vital to daily functioning and should not be taken for granted.

Balancing Occupational Roles for Optimal Health

The optimally healthy individual exhibits a finely tuned balance of the occupational areas of work, self-care, play and leisure, rest, and sleep (Figure 3–2). This individual can function more than adequately on a daily basis. The healthy individual is able to balance the five aspects of occupation and knows how to efficiently fit these into the 24 hours that we are allotted each day. When these five aspects of our lives fall out of sync and become unbalanced, we have what is known in the profession as a "problem."

In today's fast-paced and hectic lifestyle, however, most of us do not achieve this balance. Today's lifestyle norm requires us to put most of our efforts into work. There is even a coined term for this: workaholic. The majority of a person's energy goes into his work, to the exclusion of other activities (Figure 3–3). We praise this person for "burning the midnight oil" or "burning the candle at both ends." However, continuing to work at this kind of pace, over a sustained period of time, often leads these so-called "supermen" and "superwomen" to eventually burn out and become ill, either physically or psychologically.

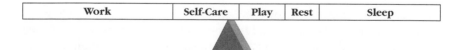

Work	Self-Care	Play	Rest	Sleep

Figure 3-2. The healthy individual. All occupational role performance areas (work, self-care, play/leisure, rest, and sleep) are in optimal balance.

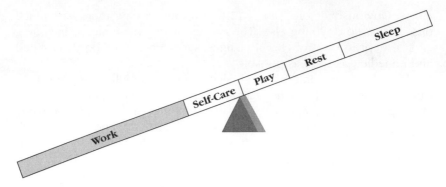

Figure 3-3. The workaholic. Too much emphasis on work throws other role performance areas out of balance.

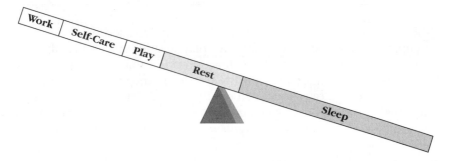

Figure 3-4. The person with an illness or disability. Work and self-care are replaced with too much rest, sleep, and forced leisure time.

On the other hand, when one does become ill, disabled, incapacitated, or even chronically unemployed, the balance shifts the other way (Figure 3–4). In this scenario, work diminishes and is overcompensated by forced rest and sleep. In the case of illness, play becomes nonexistent, and self-care needs may have to be addressed by others. Once again, the balance is gone.

What about children? They don't work—isn't their balance also out of whack? As you may recall, I said that play is a child's work. Most of their time is consumed with play. Young children have most of their self-care needs met by others, and another large segment of their time is concerned with rest and sleep (Figure 3–5). As children grow older and enter school, this balance again shifts, with an increase in independent self-care skills and schoolwork displacing some of the children's playtime.

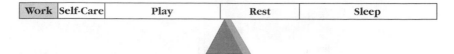

Work	Self-Care	Play	Rest	Sleep

Figure 3-5. Children spend the majority of their time involved in play. Play is the antecedent to work. Play also helps children to learn rules, skills, and roles in a safe, nonthreatening atmosphere.

Time Management Skills

Closely related to balancing occupational roles each day is time management, or temporal adaptation. In order to be healthy and effective in day-to-day activities, it is essential to be able to use time effectively, rather than be used by time (or, in essence, be a slave to time). People who do not know how to use time well are constantly "behind the eight ball," or they may become bored and lose the desire to try to effectively utilize time altogether.

In any given 24-hour time period, we must accomplish a certain number of things. For the sake of argument, we will assume that one-third, or eight hours, of our time will be spent asleep. This leaves us 16 hours to accomplish everything else we need to do. If we get up at 7:00 A.M. and spend one hour getting ready for work, one hour traveling to work, eight hours at work, and one hour coming home, we should be home by 6:00 P.M. (Figure 3–6). We now have five hours all to ourselves to do whatever we want! But wait. You may have to make dinner, clean up, pay bills, catch up on some paperwork, walk the dog, and check the mail. If you have children, you have to supervise them, including helping with homework, getting ready for bed, monitoring television, computer, or video game use, and reading books. I don't know about you, but I'm exhausted!

Can you imagine what life would be like if you were not a master of time management? Well, there are plenty of people who are not. These individuals do not use time effectively, and, in fact, they are frequently used by time. These are the people who never seem to have enough time to get things done. They rush around, constantly doing things, and yet they never seem to accomplish anything. Poor time-management skills can lead to anxiety, depression, procrastination, frustration, anger, and diminished interpersonal and occupational interactions. Other than that, it's no big deal.

For example, the average working adult can usually get himself up in the morning, shower, dress, eat, and get to work. Self-care is no problem. That same person may put in a 12-hour workday, come home exhausted,

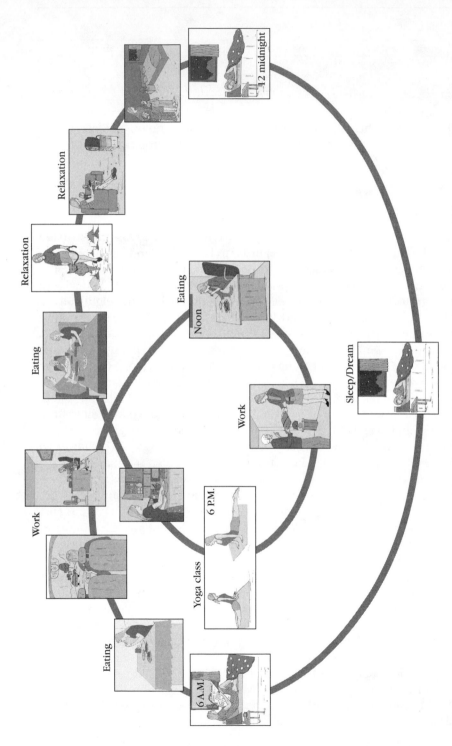

Figure 3-6. Circadian rhythms provide a built-in, biological scheduling system. When these rhythms are interfered with, daily functioning can be severely impaired.

Relaxation

Relaxation

Eating

Eating

Noon

Work

Work

Sleep/Dream

6 P.M.

Yoga class

Eating

6 A.M.

12 midnight

struggle to take care of things around the house, get to bed around 11:30 P.M., and start the next day at 5:00 A.M. This continues every day, ad nauseum. You may have noticed that there is no room for play and leisure activities, or what Steven Covey refers to as "sharpening the saw" in *The Seven Habits of Highly Successful People* (p. 287). If he has no release from this endless drudgery, he will experience physical or mental health problems down the road. All work and no play makes Jack a dull boy. All work and no play makes Jack a dull boy. All work and no play makes Jack a dull boy. (oops! Sorry, I've been watching *The Shining* again).

How Occupational Therapy Helps People

George Barton (1915), one of the founders of the profession, once posed the question: "If there are occupational diseases, why not occupational therapy?" Barton, himself disabled, believed that occupation held the key to all diseases and disabilities, and he passionately pursued this **paradigm,** or model, throughout his life.

The essence of occupational therapy is twofold: using occupation to restore function and enabling the patient to pursue occupation as a result of therapy. Confusing? Not really. Let's take a look.

As I have already stated, we all use occupation every day. Therefore, using occupation as a means to rehabilitate, or even to habilitate, makes a great deal of sense. Physically participating in any activity takes a certain amount of skill, dexterity, coordination, strength, endurance, and sensory awareness. Rather than try to increase a person's strength and dexterity merely with exercise, the occupational therapist uses occupation to meet those goals and more, resulting in a tangible product or skill.

At the same time, using occupation as therapy can allow the individual to effectively perform that activity when therapy comes to an end. Furthermore, the mastering of one occupational skill can frequently help an individual to perform and master other occupations that are important to her.

For example, Mrs. Jones is a 68-year-old homemaker who has recently suffered a stroke, which has paralyzed her right side. She is no longer able to use her dominant right arm and hand, and she can no longer cook, clean, shop, work in her beloved flower garden, or do things such as bathe, dress, and feed herself.

The occupational therapist first determines the extent of Mrs. Jones's deficits and notes her residual strengths, both physical and emotional.

The therapist then identifies her interests and uses these interests to develop a therapy program that may or may not include the following:

1. Work with Mrs. Jones's right arm and hand in order to normalize muscle tone, preserve range of motion, and facilitate the return of strength and fine motor skills.

2. Teach Mrs. Jones to perform activities such as dressing, bathing, grooming, meal preparation, and housecleaning in alternate ways, such as by using her left hand to perform activities, her right hand and arm to assist, and instructing her in the use of appropriate assistive devices to perform activities.

3. Graduate or grade each activity, from easy to more difficult, in order to challenge Mrs. Jones without overwhelming and frustrating her.

4. Educate Mrs. Jones and her husband in ways to adapt her garden to make it easier for her to continue to participate in this important area of her life.

It should be noted that each of these goals addresses a different occupational performance for Mrs. Jones. Because she is a homemaker, this is her job and her work. Therefore, the goals that address meal preparation and housework are geared toward the worker portion of her personality.

The self-care goals are self evident. Most people do not really want other people to help them with self-care activities unless they absolutely cannot do them on their own. Finally, although gardening would feel like work to me, Mrs. Jones finds this relaxing and pleasurable and, therefore, to her it is a leisure activity (and an important one, at that).

As Mrs. Jones achieves each of these goals, a new goal may be developed to replace it. If she should fail to meet a goal, the therapist must revisit and revise the goal, in order to make it more achievable (goals will be discussed in more detail in Chapter 7).

SUMMARY

This chapter has focused on presenting basic concepts of occupational therapy and defining the component parts that make up occupation—work, self-care, play and leisure, rest, and sleep—and the balance between these components that is essential to physical and mental health. The concepts of temporal adaptation and time management were also discussed, as they relate to occupational role balance and performance. Finally, this chapter described the functional application of these concepts to real-life occupational therapy practice and provided an example for the reader.

References

Barton, G. (1915). Occupational therapy. *Trained Nurse Hospital Review, 54,* 138–140.

Cawood, L. T. (1975). *WORDS: Work-oriented rehabilitation dictionary and synonyms.* Seattle, WA: Northwest Association of Rehabilitation Industries.

Covey, S. (1989). *The seven habits of highly successful people: Powerful lessons in personal change.* New York: Simon & Schuster.

Deloach, C., & Greer, B. (1981). *Adjustments to serve physical disability: A metamorphosis.* New York: McGraw-Hill.

Merriam-Webster's new collegiate dictionary (3rd ed.). (1973). Springfield, MA: Merriam-Webster.

Mosey, A. C. (1973). *Activities therapy.* New York: Raven Press.

Reilly, M. (1974). Play as exploratory learning. Beverly Hills, CA: Sage Publications.

Shannon, P. D. (1970). Work adjustment and the adolescent soldier. *American Journal of Occupational Therapy, 24,* 112.

Trombly, C. A. (1995). *Occupational therapy for physical dysfunction* (4th ed.). Baltimore, MD: Williams & Wilkins.

CHAPTER 4

Occupational Therapy Education

Chapter Goals

At the conclusion of this chapter, the reader should:

- Know the educational requirements of an occupational therapist, registered (OTR).

- Know the educational requirements of a certified occupational therapy assistant (COTA).

- Have a basic understanding of the concepts of illness and wellness.

- Have a basic understanding of the concepts of research, ethics, theory, and clinical reasoning, as they apply to occupational therapy practice.

INTRODUCTION

Becoming an occupational therapist is easy. All one has to do is locate, apply to, and be accepted by an accredited occupational therapy (OT) program; do the required work, pass everything, and graduate; and pass the national examination. No problem.

To be a good occupational therapist, on the other hand, requires all of that educational stuff plus a handful of other qualifications, including life experience, empathy, good people skills, and a sense of humor. You should have known that there would be a catch!

In this chapter, we will look at all of these requirements and explore how they fit together to form the big picture.

Educational Requirements

Before we begin this part of our exploration, we must familiarize ourselves with the two levels of occupational therapy practice: entry-level practitioners, or OTRs, and technical-level practitioners, or COTAs. Each of these levels has its own educational requirements, and these will present cost differences.

One must invest a minimum of five years of college in order to receive an entry-level master's of occupational therapy degree (MOT). The occupational therapy assistant route (a noble path, I might add, as that is where I began my own career) requires two years of college and yields an associate of applied science degree (AAS), although there are a few one-year certificate programs still available.

So what's the difference, you ask? Why not go to school for two years instead of five? Good question; let us now look at the differences between the two routes.

There are 161 entry-level OT programs accredited by the Accreditation Council for Occupational Therapy Education (ACOTE) in the United States. These are located in 43 states within the continental United States, with two in Puerto Rico. A degree from one of these fine institutions, and subsequent passing of the National Registration Examination administered by the National Board for Certification in Occupational Therapy (NBCOT), allows the graduate to become an OTR.

An OTR is able, with a physician's order, to perform complete occupational therapy evaluations, draw up treatment plans, and treat clients— essentially, she can do anything necessary within the scope of occupational therapy practice. An OTR has more autonomy than a COTA (which I will get to in a minute) and can work anywhere she finds a niche. An OTR is often placed in supervisory roles, and management positions are common for those with advanced degrees.

Occupational therapists also make more money than COTAs; the U.S. Department of Labor cites the current average salary for an occupational therapist as approximately $55,000. This, of course, will vary depending on geographic location and specialty area of practice. For example, a therapist working in an urban rehabilitation center is probably going to command a higher salary than one who is working a nine-month schedule in a suburban school district.

Of course, becoming a COTA is a good idea, too. Personally, I began my career as a COTA and have no regrets about it. In fact, I believe that I am a much better therapist for having pursued my career in this manner. If I had initially gone to a four-year school, there is a very good chance that I would have flunked out or quit, and I wouldn't be writing this book now.

By pursuing the COTA route, I had a chance to try on the occupational therapist role in a relatively quick (two years) and inexpensive way. If, at the end of that time, I decided that I didn't like it, I was free to go on to something else; at least I had a degree. I have been very fortunate, however, in that I not only love what I do, but I really believe that I was born to do this work.

People often ask me why I carried on with my occupational therapy education. For me, the reason was strictly financial. Back in 1978, my first job paid $6,500 a year and, after a few years, my annual salary maxed out at just over $10,000. I could not afford to live on that salary, so I was forced to continue my education. I should point out that, today, COTAs make much better salaries. I am also a very nontraditional, nonconformist individual. I tend to be very independent, and my two-year degree did not allow as much latitude as I desired in my employment situation.

Having bored you with that bunch of useless trivia, let me say that there are many COTAs, if not the vast majority, who remain COTAs throughout their careers and would have it no other way. This is a good thing, too, because there is a great need for COTAs in today's health care market.

So what does a COTA do? A COTA does pretty much all of the things that an OTR does, with a few exceptions, but is supervised by an OTR. A COTA cannot perform an autonomous occupational therapy evaluation and can only carry out certain aspects of the evaluation process under the direction of, or in conjunction with, the OTR.

Perhaps the biggest limitation for COTAs is that they need to be supervised by an OTR on a regular basis. On the upside, however, they get to spend more hands-on time with clients and have less paperwork to worry about (although one can never fully escape the dreaded paperwork).

There are 139 occupational therapy assistant (OTA) programs accredited by ACOTE in the United States, including schools in 41 states within the continental United States (where both my alma mater and current employer are located), one in Hawaii (aloha!), and one in Puerto Rico (buenos dias!). Again, most OTA programs are two years in length and, in addition to the core occupational therapy courses, include other areas like anatomy and physiology, English, and social sciences. Math is usually not a major prerequisite (which is one of the reasons why I am an occupational therapist).

According to www.collegegrad.com, COTAs held about 18,000 jobs in 2002, with an average salary of $36,000. This is not a bad salary for a two-year investment, and it has certainly come a long way since I was a COTA!

Courses of Study

Once a student has been accepted into an accredited occupational therapy program, what courses of study will she take? This section will provide a basic overview, although every school will differ in the exact courses it offers. Furthermore, those going for an associates degree will take different courses than those going for a more advanced degree.

Let us imagine the total course content shaped like a pyramid (Figure 4–1). A pyramid has a very wide and stable base of support and

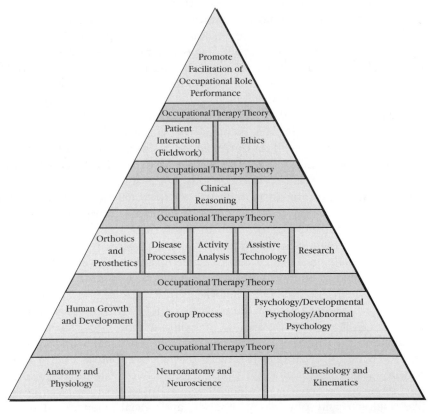

Figure 4-1. Occupational therapy educational pyramid

becomes narrower as it approaches the apex, or endpoint. I will present the course work, or the foundation of the profession, in this manner. The order of the presentation is somewhat subjective, but I believe that it makes good sense in terms of building upon a strong framework.

We begin with **anatomy** and **physiology,** because a good understanding of the human body and how it works is essential if we are to rehabilitate physical problems. Knowledge of the bones and muscles, as well as the cardiopulmonary system, will impact the effectiveness of treatment.

Closely associated with anatomy are **neuroanatomy** and **neuroscience.** As complicated as the brain and nervous system are, and as much as we still do not know about them, there is a semblance of order to the arrangement. The occupational therapist and occupational therapy assistant must be be familiar with their structures and functions. The art of rehabilitation emerges from this basic knowledge, in the form of neuro-developmental training, Bobath techniques, reflex-inhibiting positioning, and sensory integration.

Another important area of study is **kinesiology,** the study of movement. It is one thing to know the names of the muscles and the physiology of how they work, but it is also important to understand what movements the primary movers (**agonists**) perform, which muscles work with them (**synergists**), and which muscles work against them (**antagonists**). A bit of basic physics is involved in this course, in order to give students a good understanding of movement.

Closely associated with kinesiology is the ability to measure muscle strength and joint movement. Muscle strength is typically measured using a quasi-objective rating system known as the Manual Muscle Test (Figure 4–2). Another muscle-strength test is performed using an instrument known as a **dynamometer** (*dyn* means force), which is more **objective** in its findings and serves as a fairly accurate device. Dynamometers are typically used to test manual grip and pinch strength, but they can also be used to test other muscle groups (Figure 4–3).

Joint movement is tested using an instrument known as a **goniometer** (Figure 4–4). This allows the therapist to measure joint range of motion prior to beginning therapy and to perform intermittent measurements to determine any changes in joint movement. The goniometer is a simple-looking instrument, but it takes practice to increase one's expertise with it.

Moving from the physical to the psychological and emotional aspects of the client, the courses of study include, in ascending order, psychology, abnormal psychiatry, and occupational therapy as it applies to psychosocial impairments.

Psychology provides a basic understanding of what makes people tick. The major theorists, such as **Sigmund Freud, Carl Jung, Carl Rogers,**

5	Normal	N	The body part moves through full range of motion against maximum resistance and gravity.
4	Good	G	The body part moves through full range of motion against gravity and moderate resistance.
	Fair plus	F+	The body part moves through full range of motion against gravity and minimal resistance.
3	Fair	F	The body part moves through full range of motion with no added resistance.
	Fair minus	F−	The body part moves through less-than-full range of motion against gravity.
	Poor plus	P+	The body part moves through full range of motion with gravity eliminated and then relaxes suddenly.
2	Poor	P	The body part moves through full range of motion with gravity eliminated and with no added resistance.
	Poor minus	P−	The body part moves through less-than-full range of motion with gravity eliminated.
1	Trace	T	Tension can be felt in the muscle but no movement occurs.
0	Zero	0	No muscle tension can be detected.

Adapted from Trombly, C. A. (1995). *Occupational therapy for physical dysfunction* (4th ed.). Baltimore, MD: Williams & Wilkins.

Figure 4-2. The Manual Muscle Test (MMT) is the most common method used by therapists to evaluate muscle strength.

Ivan Pavlov, and **B. F. Skinner,** are studied, as well as others. Students learn about the **id, ego, superego, behaviorism,** and **conditioned response,** along with other basic psychological concepts.

Abnormal psychiatry focuses on the aberrant conditions of the human psyche, such as **depression, bipolar disease, schizophrenia, anxiety disorders,** and **personality disorders,** as well as the treatments for these conditions—both past and present.

Finally, students study the role of occupational therapy in working with these conditions. As you may recall, occupational therapy has its roots in psychiatry, and this tradition continues. Regardless of the area in which any occupational therapist may find himself, there will always be a psychosocial component. Because we profess to be holistic in approach, we cannot divorce the psychosocial aspects of care from the rest. Specifically, this course will examine the unique role that the occupational therapist may play when working with people struggling with

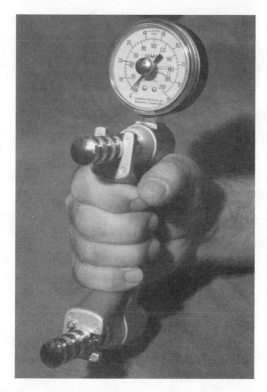

Figure 4 3. The dynamometer is an instrument used to test hand-grip strength using objective measurements that can be easily replicated by different therapists.

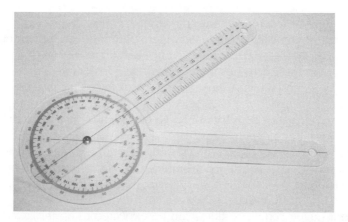

Figure 4-4. The goniometer is a device that can accurately measure the range of motion in joints.

depression, schizophrenia, substance abuse problems, and personality disorders. Let's face it: a person with schizophrenia can have a stroke too, and any physical disability can bring on a raging episode of depression. Therefore, it's a good idea to understand these conditions and know how to deal with them.

Years ago, an occupational therapy student was observing me in my home health practice. At one point, she said to me, "You're really into that psychosocial stuff, aren't you?" After recovering from my initial shock at this statement, I replied, "Yeah, I guess I am." I then went on to bore her with a long lecture on exactly why I was "really into it" and why it is so important to the overall treatment process. I hope that she has taken that lesson to heart.

A related course is the study of **group dynamics.** This course usually focuses on the interaction between two people, called **dyads** (usually the therapist and one client), and small groups generally composed of no more than 10 people. Different aspects of group behavior are examined, and group roles such as **leader, facilitator,** and **gatekeeper** are addressed. This is an important class because we all have to deal with other people, and occupational therapists often treat groups of people as well as individuals.

Therapeutic media is a broad area of study that is central to the profession of occupational therapy. This can include learning activities such as knitting, crocheting, sewing, and basketry. It may also include ceramics, woodworking, copper tooling, and mosaic tiling, or even more modern media, such as the use of computers. These activities are the tools of our trade and are frequently used with clients to promote rehabilitation, health, and wellness.

My father used to deride college courses that were outside the traditional "three Rs" (reading, writing, and arithmetic) as "basket weaving 101." I took great joy in calling him up during my junior year and announcing that I was, in fact, taking basket weaving—and it was required!

As trivial as these activities may seem, there is a method to the madness. The activities chosen by the therapist must be selected for a specific reason and must be related to the client's treatment plan. To achieve this, we use what is known as an **activity analysis;** each activity it dissected and reduced to its component elements, including age and gender appropriateness, the client's interests and desires, and the realistic expectations of actually performing the activity. Trombley (2002) stated that activity analysis "is one of the key process skills of occupational therapists. Occupational therapists analyze an activity because they want to know (1) whether the client, given certain abilities, can be expected to do the activity and (2) whether the activity can challenge latent abilities or capacities and thereby improve these" (p. 262).

For example, let's take a look at the activity of basket weaving. This seems like an easy activity, but—if we break it down—we find that it is actually quite complicated. We need to look at numerous factors in order to make a basket, including the amount of required muscle strength, the amount of sensation in the fingers and hands, the range of motion in the arms, how much vision is needed, and so on. Other factors that need to be taken into account include cultural components; that is, is this activity socially acceptable to the individual performing it, and does the individual want to perform this activity in the first place?

Another course of study common to most occupational therapy curricula is **human growth and development.** This class, or group of classes, follows human development from birth through adulthood and old age. Much of the focus is typically on the early years of childhood, and, in addition to physical changes, the psychosocial aspects of development are addressed. Developmental theorists, such as Jean Piaget, Erik Erickson, and Harry Stack Sullivan, are also addressed. This information is important because effective occupational therapy intervention must take into account the developmental level of the individual client.

Orthotics, Prosthetics, and Assistive Technology

As our educational pyramid continues to ascend, we add courses in **orthotics, prosthetics,** and **assistive technology.** Orthoses are devices designed to immobilize a body part or to facilitate function. Deshaies (2002) defined an orthosis as "any medical device added to a person's body to support, align, position, immobilize, prevent or correct deformities, assist weak muscles, or improve function" (p. 314). These devices are more commonly referred to as splints or braces.

Orthotics were originally complicated contraptions made from metal and leather, held in place by straps and buckles. Most modern orthoses are made from some type of low-temperature thermoplastic material that can be heated (to make it more pliable), molded to the affected body part, and allowed to cool, thus returning it to its original firmness. These are usually held in place by Velcro® straps.

Splints can either be static or dynamic in nature. A static splint is a fairly simple design used to immobilize a joint or body part. Static, of course, means stationary; therefore, when you splint a broken bone, you immobilize it. This type of splint can be used with broken bones, to immobilize a joint following surgery, or to help relieve the pain of arthritis.

A dynamic splint, on the other hand, is usually a simple hinge or pulley system that allows limited movement designed to promote function. An example of this is a **tenodesis splint,** which allows people with C6–C7 cervical spinal cord injuries, quadriplegics, and those who do not have finger movement (but who can actively extend their wrists) to grasp objects by a natural phenomenon known as tenodesis. When you actively or passively flex your wrist, you may notice that your fingers tend to extend and open; this makes it easy to let go of things but not to hold onto them. When you extend your wrist, you may also notice that your fingers have a tendency to flex slightly. This concept is used quite frequently in aikido and other forms of the martial arts. The tenodesis splint allows the user to grasp and release objects while wearing the splint.

Prosthetics is one of the world's oldest professions, to which Captain Hook and Peg Leg Pete can attest. A prosthesis is a device used to replace a body part either for function, cosmetic reasons, or both. A familiar example of a functional prosthesis is an artificial leg or arm, and dentures are also included in this category (although they fit into the cosmetic category, as well). Examples of cosmetic prostheses include artificial eyeballs, breasts (following a **mastectomy**), and testicles (following an **orchiectomy**). For the record, occupational therapists usually deal with artificial arms and hands. We also deal with dentures, in terms of putting them in, taking them out, and keeping them clean.

Prosthetic arms can be controlled by straps that are sensitive to certain arm movements, or they may be myoelectric. Myoelectric prostheses are innervated by electrodes that are placed over nerves and react to the user's own nerve impulses. Pretty amazing stuff—*RoboCop* wasn't too far fetched, after all! Although prosthetics are manufactured and fitted by a prosthetist, the occupational therapist is typically the one who teaches the user how to perform daily activities while wearing it.

Assistive Technology

Assistive technology, sometimes called adaptive equipment, are items that help people with disabilities to carry out everyday activities independently and easily. Examples of assistive devices can range from something as simple as increasing the diameter of a fork to allow someone with arthritis or muscle weakness to hold it and feed himself, to something as high tech as using a puff-and-sip switch to operate a power wheelchair by merely blowing into and sucking on a tube, or operating an environmental control system from a bed or wheelchair.

Physical Agent Modalities

More occupational therapy students have been educated in the use of **physical agent modalities** (PAMs) in recent years. These modalities include the use of heat and cold, paraffin, ultrasound, and electrical stimulation (e-stim). These were traditionally within the purview of physical therapists (PTs); however, a gradual blending of certain aspects of the two professions has taken place, and occupational therapists are beginning to utilize PAMs in greater numbers. Although the modalities used by occupational therapists and PTs may be the same, the reasons for their use differ. The American Occupational Therapy Association (AOTA), in its *Physical Agent Modality Position Paper* (1997), stated that

> *Physical agent modalities may be used by occupational therapy practitioners when used as an adjunct to or in preparation for purposeful activity to enhance occupational performance and when applied by a practitioner who has documented evidence of possessing the theoretical background and technical skills for safe and competent integration of the modality into an occupational therapy intervention plan. (p. 871)*

The AOTA (1997) defines physical agent modalities as "those modalities that produce a response in soft tissue through the use of light, water, temperature, sound, or electricity. Physical agent modalities include, but are not limited to, paraffin baths, hot packs, cold packs, fluidotherapy, contrast baths, ultrasound, whirlpool, and electrical stimulation units" (p. 870). Let's look at each one of these in turn.

Paraffin baths are simply liquid paraffin (wax) used to provide heat to small joints, usually those of the hands and feet. They are frequently used to relieve the pain of arthritis, whereby the affected hand (or foot) is quickly dipped into the liquid paraffin and allowed to dry. This process is repeated multiple times in order to layer the paraffin and provide more heat. The hand is then wrapped in a plastic bag, which is left on for about 20 minutes. Typically, some type of skin oil is mixed with the paraffin to help it peel off easily. A byproduct of this treatment is that it makes the skin nice and smooth; you'll be the envy of everyone on your block! With the pain relieved (albeit temporarily), the client is better able to participate in functional activities.

Hot packs (also known as hydrocollator packs) are thick pads that are heated in a **hydrocollator** to temperatures of 104–113° F (Bracciano & Earley, 2002) and usually applied to larger areas. Hot packs are really hot, so knowledge of their safe use is extremely important.

The use of cold packs, also known as **cryotherapy** (so named because most people cry during use—just kidding; actually, cryo means cold), serves to relieve pain and swelling, or edema. As you may remember from your basic first aid class, you should always apply cold temperatures to a sprain. Why? Because this prevents swelling.

Contrast baths involve the simple process of going from very warm water to very cool water, in order to relieve pain. By doing this, the pain centers in the brain become confused, and it doesn't know what to think anymore. Actually, this technique promotes a pumping action that increases blood flow, thus reducing swelling and, therefore, pain.

Fluidotherapy (Figure 4–5) uses finely ground corn husks suspended in warm air (105–118° F) and blown all around the affected extremity, a process that provides pain relief while simultaneously allowing for range of motion (Bracciano & Earley, 2002). It sounds messy, but it all takes place within a closed unit in which the client inserts his or her hand. You really must experience this to fully appreciate it.

All of the above modalities are known as **superficial heating agents** (SHAs) because they are applied to the skin and act upon the superficial tissues. These are also known as **superficial physical agent modalities** (SPAMs), which are not to be confused with the pseudo-meat product in a can or with those horrible, unwanted e-mails. Two modalities work at an even deeper level: therapeutic ultrasound and electrotherapy.

Therapeutic ultrasound produces deep heating through the use of ultrasonic waves that cause heat energy to accumulate in the deep soft tissues. This can reduce pain and promote healing, as well as facilitate function (Bracciano, 1999).

Electrotherapy involves the use of electricity to achieve a number of goals, including pain control, muscle facilitation, and edema reduction, among others. Types of electrotherapy include neuromuscular electrical

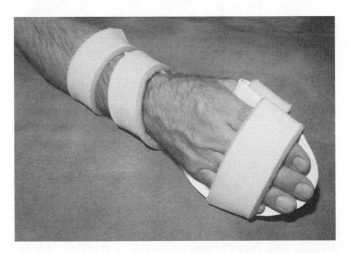

Figure 4-5. A hand splint is used to immobilize a joint or body part, or to enhance the function of a weak or paralyzed body part.

stimulation (NMES), **transcutaneous electric nerve stimulation** (TENS), **functional electrical stimulation** (FES), **electrical muscle stimulation** (EMS), and **iontophoresis** (Bracciano & Earley, 2002). Bracciano and Earley (2002) described each of these types in more detail:

- NMES uses pulsating alternating current to activate muscles through stimulation of intact peripheral nerves to cause a motor response. Stimulation of the nerve is used to decrease muscle spasm, for muscle strengthening, and for its effect on muscle pumping, which can reduce edema. NMES can also be used for muscle reeducation and to prevent atrophy.

- FES is neuromuscular facilitation to activate targeted muscle groups for orthotic substitution or to facilitate performance of functional activities. FES is often used with individuals who have shoulder subluxation or drop foot after a stroke.

- TENS describes the wide variety of stimulators used for pain control. TENS uses surface electrodes with the goal of sensory analgesia rather than a motor response.

- EMS is electrical stimulation for denevated muscle to facilitate viability and to prevent atrophy, degeneration, and fibrosis of the fibers. EMS may facilitate nerve regeneration and muscle reinnervation while decreasing muscle atrophy.

- Iontophoresis is the use of low-voltage direct currents to ionize topically applied medication into the tissue. Iontophoresis is often used in the treatment of inflammatory conditions or for scar formation and management. (p. 431)

Illness and Wellness

Classes focus on the diseases that can affect people and outline the signs and symptoms of those diseases, as well as the medical treatments available and how occupational therapy can intervene in order to help the person pursue occupation despite the disease. These diseases include multiple sclerosis, Guillain-Barré syndrome, cancer, diabetes, heart disease, chronic obstructive pulmonary disease (COPD), and arthritis, to name but a few. The diseases included are physical as well as psychiatric, and the course of study usually covers diseases across the life span, from birth through terminal illness and death. In order to deal with a disease process, one must first understand it. As martial artist Bruce Lee said in the 1973 film *Enter the Dragon,* "Never take your eyes off of your opponent."

A related subject area is the promotion of health, or **wellness.** To promote wellness, as opposed to illness, in our clients is to educate them about living a healthy lifestyle. This includes the usual subjects, such as diet and exercise, regular medical checkups, and similar areas. In today's modern world, however, it includes education on the use of moderation in habits such as nicotine, alcohol, and recreational drug use. Wellness may also include educating clients on safer sex techniques, such as condom use or abstinence, in order to avoid contracting sexually transmitted diseases (STDs), including HIV, hepatitis, chlamydia, and, of course, good old-fashioned syphilis and gonorrhea.

In addition to the above items, occupational therapy's primary focus on wellness should include striking a good balance between work, self-care, play and leisure, and rest and sleep, and the performance of beneficial occupations in everyday life. This is what the profession is about, after all.

Research, Ethics, Theory, and Clinical Reasoning

Entry-level occupational therapy students (bachelor's- or master's-degree level) will most likely take at least one course in research methods and techniques (OTA students usually don't have to contend with this). Research is important in any profession, because it defines the job and provides evidence to justify its importance to the world. Portney and Watkins (2000) stated that "Clinical research is a structured process of investigating facts and theories. It is a method of answering questions in a systematic and objective way to examine clinical conditions and outcomes, to establish relationships among clinical phenomena, and to provide the impetus for improving methods of practice" (p. 4). Research requires a working knowledge of statistics in order to carry out research studies (sorry about that). There are some therapists who love to do research and spend their careers doing just that. Bless their hearts!

Near the top of our pyramid is the study of **ethics.** This is an important topic in any field; however, when you are constantly interacting with other human beings on an intimate level, the study of ethics becomes paramount. Ethics are closely related to research, in that researchers must be wary of being unethical in the types of research they perform.

Ethics refer to the study of morality: what is right and what is wrong. Ethics have always been important to society, but they have come under greater scrutiny in recent years, both in politics and medicine. Perhaps the most important concept of ethics is the call to "do no harm" in the treatment of a client. Ultimately, the occupational therapy practitioner must always do the right thing when it comes to interacting with and treating a client in a professional relationship.

Finally, the cement that holds all of this information together is occupational therapy theory. A theoretical base is important, because it allows the practitioner to organize her intervention (Sabonis-Chafee & Hussey, 1998). Occupational therapy theory builds upon the bricks of knowledge gained from all of the courses of study within the occupational therapy curriculum and binds them together into a strong, solid structure. It draws on the knowledge base of the moral treatment movement, all the way through to the research of the 20th and 21st centuries.

Although many students roll their eyes when they hear the term *theory*, the practitioner needs to have some understanding of, and theoretical basis for, what he is doing. Crepeau and Schell (2003) stated that "theory is particularly important for new practitioners who have little experience to draw on" (p. 206). Ottenbacher (cited in Crepeau & Schell, 2003) stated that theory is "most useful when it helps a therapist predict what will occur in treatment" (p. 205). Without a theoretical base, therapists might frequently apply the balloon approach to therapy—that is, blowing up a balloon and letting it go without really having an idea of where it will land. In essence, theory keeps us grounded and focused.

The theoretical framework is addressed in all occupational therapy programs, but greater emphasis is placed on theory in the entry-level programs. Entry-level therapists are expected to build upon the theoretical base, while occupational therapy assistants are technicians who execute treatment plans in their purest forms.

Closely related to theory, and incorporating all of this newly acquired knowledge, is the concept of **clinical reasoning.** According to Schell (2003), "Clinical reasoning is the process used by practitioners to plan, direct, perform, and reflect on client care" (p. 131). Punwar and Peloquin (2000) stated that clinical reasoning allows the therapist to "make judgments based on observation, knowledge and experience. By drawing on his or her accumulated experience, a therapist is often able to know which goals may be most important to the client and which therapeutic activities may have the most meaning" (p. 103).

Mattingly and Flemming (1994) argued that the concept of clinical reasoning is complex and defies a simple definition or explanation (which is apparently why they wrote an entire book about it). They believed that

> *To talk about how therapists think is necessarily to consider what therapists think about, what they perceive in the way they view their clients, what they focus on as the central problem, what they ignore, how they describe what is physiologically problematic for the client, and even their view of who the client is as a person. (p. 9)*

Lewin and Reed (1998) posited that "effective therapists need to think beyond what is" (p. 5) and essentially think outside of the box and see the big picture in all its panoramic, sensorial glory. In a nutshell, clinical reasoning involves looking at the client as a unique person and determining exactly how the utilized treatment method will impact him as an individual. Clinical reasoning is ultimately hard to define and can only be intuited by years of clinical experience; it has been said that clinical reasoning cannot be taught, but it can be learned. In a way, this is similar to a runner or athlete who is in "the zone"—the concept is difficult to explain until one actually experiences it.

Fieldwork and the Real World

Upon completion of all of the didactic classroom stuff, students are released into the real world and spend the last few months of their education in supervised clinical fieldwork placements. It should be noted that they do get a small taste of the real world in level I placements; however, the final phase, or level II clinicals, is what separates the wheat from the chaff. Typically, the student performs two separate placements in two different types of clinical settings. For the technical-level occupational therapy assistant student, each clinical is 8 weeks long, while each clinical is 12 weeks long for the entry-level student. Some schools require three placements, but most only require two.

The student gets to work with "real" people during these clinicals, and she gets to apply all of her book knowledge (or what she can remember) to real-world experiences. This can be, and usually is, a terrifying prospect for the student who feels as though she is constantly under the microscope. One of my students once said to me, "You know, no matter how much you read, listen to lectures, or take tests, nothing can prepare you for the real thing." She was absolutely right!

Upon successful completion of all course work and clinical assignments, the student graduates. She is then eligible to take either the certification examination or the registration examination (both of which are offered by NBCOT), which allow the successful applicant to become a COTA or an OTR, respectively.

As the general population ages, particularly the baby boomers, the health care industry will continue to expand exponentially. This growth will include all allied health professions, especially occupational therapy. Employment for both OTRs and COTAs is expected to grow at a rate faster than average, for all occupations, through the year 2012 (www.collegegrad.com).

Traits Necessary to Be an Effective Therapist

Not everyone has the necessary skills to be a good and effective occupational therapist. In addition to grasping all of the educational basics, the most important quality one needs to possess is good people skills. If the therapist cannot connect with the client, the therapeutic relationship is lost, and the therapist may not be able to get the most out of the client. Let's examine some of the traits that contribute to a good therapist.

The Emotional Intelligence Factor

It has long been my personal contention that being a good occupational therapist requires much more than merely getting good grades. In fact, by anecdotal observation, I have noted that those students who are ac-ademically superior are frequently, in my humble opinion, the worst therapists. Although being "book smart" is important in any profession, there are many other important factors to consider. Daniel Goleman (1995) referred to these traits as *emotional intelligence*, which includes effectively reading other people, getting along with others, self-awareness, impulse control, persistence, and having a well-developed sense of empathy.

Although emotional intelligence is important in almost any aspect of life, it is paramount when you are working with at-risk individuals on a daily basis. An important aspect of occupational therapy is facilitating the therapeutic process and encouraging your clients to do their very best. If you have poor interpersonal skills, this process is not going to go well.

Of all of the aspects of emotional intelligence, I believe that the most important one is empathy. Empathy is "the ability to understand what another person is thinking or feeling, without reactions of pity or distress" (Punwar & Peloquin, 2000, p. 96). Empathy may be innate in some, but it can be learned by most (except for sociopaths, who are incapable of empathy). However, the learning process may take years—if not a lifetime—and could involve a great deal of personal introspection and emotional pain.

One cannot be an effective occupational therapist if one does not possess a well-developed sense of empathy. I cannot be more explicit about this; if you are not an empathetic person, you will have poor results with your clients. Some people are simply more empathetic than others, which is not necessarily a bad thing—it just depends on a person's choice of profession. The occupational therapy profession, however, requires empathy.

I like to think of myself as a very empathetic person, which works well in my chosen profession of occupational therapy. However, this would not work so well if I were a police or correctional officer. My empathy would work against me in those lines of work. I would probably let criminals go, or let inmates get away with things that might endanger me or allow them to escape.

Good, effective communication skills are closely related to empathy. The majority of communication involves effective, active listening. Everyone wants to be heard, and nothing can mess up a relationship quicker than one person only half-listening and misunderstanding the other person. Has this ever happened to you? Irritating, isn't it? Effective listening isn't just a matter of common sense, it can also be a matter of *common cents*; research has shown that clients are more likely to sue physicians and other health care professionals whom they feel do not listen to them.

So, how do you convey to another person that you are actively listening to him? The answer is actually very simple: body language, acknowledgement, and clarification.

Body language implies that you are, in fact, listening to the other person, and are truly interested in what she is saying. Therefore, you need to look like you are interested. Looking interested generally requires that you assume a similar posture (i.e., if she is sitting, so are you), lean toward her, and present a facial expression that usually involves eye contact. If you are writing notes or reading the newspaper while she is talking (something men never do), you will not convey a sense of interest and, ultimately, will get little cooperation.

Acknowledgement involves simply letting the person know that you are listening to him. The best way to acknowledge the person is to repeat back what he is saying—either word for word or by paraphrasing. Repeating what he says acknowledges the fact that you are listening closely; this technique is called *mirroring*.

To clarify something means to make it clear. When you are in an active conversation with someone, you clarify what you *think* you heard him say in order to make sure you heard what he *meant* to say.

For example, if we are observing an interaction between a therapist and a new client, we might witness a scene such as this:

Therapist: "Hey, Mr. Roberts, how are you doing today?"
Client: "I'm okay, I guess."
Therapist: "You're okay, you guess?" (Mirroring/Acknowledgement)
Client: "Well, I didn't sleep too well last night."
Therapist: "You didn't sleep too well last night?" (Mirroring/Acknowledgement)
Client: "Yeah, I had some pain in my back and it kept waking me up."

Therapist: "You had some pain in your back and it kept waking you up?" (Mirroring/Acknowledgement)

Client: "That's right."

Therapist: "So, you're not really feeling all that great today because you had back pain that kept you awake last night." (Clarification)

Client: "Yeah. But my back doesn't hurt now."

Therapist: "Your back doesn't hurt right now. Do you feel up to doing some work with me?" (Acknowledgement)

Client: "Yeah, I guess I could."

Therapist: "Alright! Let's get going, then!"

By repeating back exactly what the client said, the therapist let him know that he was being heard. The therapist did this quite a bit and, if you noticed, each time she got more information from Mr. Roberts without having to pull teeth. After mirroring a few times, she then clarified what Mr. Roberts meant, to be sure that she understood him and that he felt understood.

When people feel listened to, heard, and understood, the vistas of good communication are opened, and this frequently leads to greater cooperation between both therapist and client.

Listening is usually assumed and can often be taken for granted. Most of us think of ourselves as good listeners, but the sad truth is that most of us are actually very poor at it. In the words of Simon and Garfunkel's well-known song, *The Sound of Silence*, "And in the naked light I saw 10,000 people, maybe more. People talking without speaking. People hearing without listening. . . ." Effective listening is hard work, and it takes constant practice.

SUMMARY

This chapter has presented the educational requirements for occupational therapy and occupational therapy assistant students, as well as some of the differences between the entry-level occupational therapist and the assistant. A pyramid was formed to represent the educational process with the base comprised of anatomy, neuroscience, kinesiology, psychology, group process, and human growth and development. The upper half of the pyramid included orthotics and prosthetics, disease processes, activity analysis, assistive technology, ethics, clinical reasoning, patient interaction, and promotion of occupational role performance. The concepts of emotional intelligence and effective listening skills were addressed as two of the most important traits of a good occupational therapist.

References

American Occupational Therapy Association (1997). Physical agent modalities position paper. *American Journal of Occupational Therapy. 51* (10), 870–871.

Anderson, K., Anderson, L., & Glanze, W. (Eds.). (1997). *Mosby's medical, nursing, and allied health dictionary* (5th ed.). St. Louis, MO: Mosby.

Bracciano, A. (1999). Therapeutic ultrasound: Sound information for the occupational therapist. *OT Practice, 4*(1), 20–25.

Bracciano, A., & Earley, D. (2002). Physical agent modalities. In T. A. Trombly & M. V. Radomski (Eds.), *Occupational therapy for physical dysfunction* (5th ed., pp. 421–441). Philadelphia, PA: Lippincott Williams & Wilkins.

Cameron, M. H. (1999). *Physical agents in rehabilitation from research to practice*. Philadelphia, PA: Saunders.

Crepeau, E. B., & Schell, B. A. B. (2003). Theory and practice in occupational therapy. In E. B. Crepeau, E. S. Cohn, & B. A. B. Schell (Eds.), *Willard and Spackman's occupational therapy* (10th ed., pp. 203–207). Philadelphia, PA: Lippincott Williams & Wilkins.

Deshaies, L. D. (2002). Upper extremity othoses. In C. A. Trombly & M. V. Radomski (Eds.), *Occupational therapy for physical dysfunction* (5th ed., pp. 313–349). Philadelphia, PA: Lippincott Williams & Wilkins.

Goleman, D. (1995). *Emotional intelligence: Why it can matter more than IQ*. New York: Bantam Books.

Lewin, J. E., & Reed., C. A. (1998). *Creative problem solving in occupational therapy*. Philadelphia, PA: Lippincott.

Mattingly, C., & Fleming, M. H. (1994). *Clinical reasoning: Forms of inquiry in a therapeutic practice*. Philadelphia, PA: F. A. Davis Company.

Portney, L. G., & Watkins, M. P. (2000). *Foundations of clinical research applications to practice* (2nd ed.). Upper Saddle River, NJ: Prentice Hall.

Punwar, A. J., & Peloquin, S. M. (2000). *Occupational therapy principles and practice* (3rd ed.). Baltimore, MD: Lippincott Williams & Wilkins.

Sabonis-Chafee, B., & Hussey, S. M. (1998). *Introduction to occupational therapy* (2nd ed.). St. Louis, MO: Mosby.

Schell, B. A. B. (2003). Clinical reasoning: The basis for practice. In E. B. Crepeau, E. S. Cohn, & B. A. B. Schell (Eds.), *Willard and Spackman's occupational therapy* (10th ed., pp. 313–339). Philadelphia, PA: Lippincott Williams & Wilkins.

Trombley, C. A. (2002). Occupation. In T. A. Trombly & M. V. Radomski (Eds.), *Occupational therapy for physical dysfunction* (5th ed., pp. 255–281). Philadelphia, PA: Lippincott Williams & Wilkins.

CHAPTER 5

Where Do Occupational Therapists Work?

Chapter Goals

At the conclusion of this chapter, the reader should:

- Have a basic understanding of the role of the occupational therapist and occupational therapy assistant in the psychosocial practice arena.

- Have a basic understanding of the role of the occupational therapist and occupational therapy assistant in the physical dysfunction practice arena.

- Have a basic understanding of the role of the occupational therapist and occupational therapy assistant in the pediatric and school-based practice arena.

- Have a basic understanding of the role of the occupational therapist and occupational therapy assistant in nontraditional practice arenas.

INTRODUCTION

As I mentioned in Chapter 4, the demand for occupational therapy services is high, and it will continue to grow through the year 2012 and probably beyond (www.collegegrad.com). The sites where occupational therapists can be found working are many, and new practice arenas will develop as the need for services continues to grow. This chapter will discuss the more traditional areas first, then some nontraditional areas, and will finish up with some possible future areas of practice.

Psychosocial Practice

Because occupational therapy originated in the moral treatment movement, which was heavily influenced by psychiatry, I will begin with the psychosocial arena. Psychiatric occupational therapy is truly where the profession began. Many people with psychological or emotional problems have a difficult time functioning within society and require the assistance of numerous professionals, including occupational therapists.

The psychiatric occupational therapist can assist the patient in any number of ways. One of these methods includes learning how to interact with others in a one-to-one relationship, as well as in groups. This may seem like a trivial thing, but many people are unable to relate to others. These dyads, or small group sessions, may simply involve talking, or they may revolve around an activity, such as making a craft or cooking. These sessions help the participants learn the rules and roles involved in the group dynamic, and they enable them to learn potentially helpful social skills.

Another important area is time management (Chapter 3). Many people claim to have problems with time management, but psychiatric patients have problems to such an extent that they are completely unable to function adequately, obtain and maintain a job, establish meaningful relationships, or even enjoy a hobby. The occupational therapist can assist the patient in organizing her time within a specific 24-hour schedule, to include a balance of work, self-care, play and leisure, rest, and sleep. This is what Adolf Meyer and Eleanor Clarke Slagle would have referred to as "habit training."

Other areas of occupational therapy intervention might include self-care skills training, relaxation training, and anger management training, to name just a few. These are areas that most of us take for granted. However, for people with psychological or emotional problems, these are major daily problems, and the ability to solve these problems is the focus of occupational therapy intervention.

Sadly, there are very few occupational therapists still working in the psychiatric arena. Many psychiatric specialists have retired, and younger therapists are no longer pursuing this area of practice. In fact, only about

5% of all occupational therapists work in mental health. As a result, a huge population of patients is missing out on the benefits of occupational therapy. Occupational therapists have slowly been replaced with activity and recreational therapists. I believe that there must be a renaissance of occupational therapy within the psychiatric arena if there is to be a substantial change in the way the mentally ill are treated and integrated into society.

Physical Disabilities

The profession of occupational therapy attached itself to the medical model of care in the years following World War II. As a result, the majority of practicing occupational therapy personnel can be found working in hospitals, rehabilitation centers, outpatient clinics, and home health facilities. We will examine each of these areas.

Occupational therapists who work in acute care hospitals may see a variety of conditions, including cerebral vascular accidents (CVAs) or strokes, orthopedic problems (such as fractures and joint replacements), burns, and cardiac patients. Treatment within the hospital setting is usually brief, as patients are typically discharged quickly (remember the prospective payment system?) and sent to another level of care, such as inpatient rehabilitation, outpatient rehabilitation, home health, or long-term care.

Inpatient Rehabilitation

Inpatient rehabilitation centers focus on obtaining maximum results from each patient, and patients are frequently accepted into these centers based on the perceived potential for a strong recovery. The types of patients seen here are similar to those seen in acute care hospitals: strokes, postoperative joint replacements, and stable cardiac patients. The idea is to rehabilitate them to their maximal abilities and send them home, with follow-up care from either a home health agency or an outpatient clinic. Inpatient rehabilitation tends to be very structured and intense; an inpatient may be seen by occupational therapy professionals (and others) two to three times a day, five to six days a week.

Outpatient Therapy

The outpatient clinic serves people who may not require inpatient care, and who are able to leave their homes and come to the clinic. This may include people who have already completed inpatient rehabilitation or home health programs, or people who are still active and working but require therapy for a specific problem. These problems may include hand injuries, repetitive stress disorders, residual problems from a stroke, or cardiac rehabilitation. The outpatient travels to the clinic, receives treatment, and returns home following the therapeutic session.

Many outpatient clinics offer programs in work hardening; this involves working with people who are no longer able to perform, or are having difficulty performing, their jobs. In a sense, work hardening truly is occupational therapy, in that the therapist specifically works with the client in order to return him to the work arena.

Work hardening can include muscle strengthening and endurance training to help the client be able to perform his job. Simulated work activities can be graded, from easy to difficult, at a pace that will help the client effectively perform his required job functions.

Tasks can be examined and adaptations can be recommended to facilitate successful performance. For example, in today's modern work world, many (if not most) employees use computers as part of their jobs. As a result of this increase in computer use, many people develop the repetitive stress injury commonly known as carpal tunnel syndrome (CTS; see Chapter 9). This seemingly benign condition can cause severe pain and muscle atrophy if not addressed in a timely manner. Many workers are forced to stop working, at least temporarily, until the condition is either surgically corrected or resolved on its own.

The individual with CTS may come to occupational therapy for muscle strengthening, splinting of the affected hand or hands, and modalities such as ultrasound treatment. Work hardening is also employed in order to return the client to her job as quickly as possible, with education and adaptations implemented to prevent a recurrence of the condition. To achieve this, the therapist may educate the client on better sitting postures, using back supports, and foot rests. Additionally, the therapist may recommend using wrist rests while keyboarding, or changing the traditional keyboard to an ergonomic one that puts less stress on the individual's wrists.

Home Health

Home health care caters to those patients who are not appropriate for inpatient rehabilitation but are classified as "homebound" and cannot get to outpatient therapy. The term *homebound* means that, for whatever reason, the patient is not able to easily get out of the house in order to receive treatment. This may be due to the patient being bed-bound or wheelchair-bound, being unsafe in ambulation (i.e., experiencing frequent falls), or having another condition for which leaving the home would be contraindicated (i.e., not recommended). Patients who are home-bound but unable to drive must make appropriate arrangements for transportation.

The homebound patient may need a wide variety of occupational therapy services for a wide variety of reasons. The ultimate goal of home health occupational therapy is to prepare the patient for another level of care, such as in- or outpatient care, or to maximize the patient's functions so that he can function independently and safely within the home, with or without assistance.

Long-Term Care

It is no secret that most of us will grow old. Many of us will reach a point in our lives where, due to age, accident, or disease, we will not be able to take care of ourselves easily or safely. When this occurs and there are no friends or relatives to assist us with our needs, many of us may end up in a long-term care facility.

Regardless of the type of facility, whether an assisted living facility (ALF) or a skilled nursing facility (SNF), residents may well require occupational therapy intervention. This intervention may be as simple as adapting a pen to help someone hold it and sign her name, to fabricating a splint to relieve the pain of rheumatoid arthritis. Regardless of age, everyone has the need and the right to participate in life through the practice of occupation.

Pediatrics and School Systems

Another sizable practice area for occupational therapists is pediatrics, or working with children. Sadly, not all children are born healthy and perfect. Many children, due to prenatal (occurring during pregnancy and before birth), perinatal (occurring during the birthing process), and postnatal (occurring after birth) difficulties, have developmental problems such as spina bifida, cerebral palsy, autism, mental retardation, and Asperger's syndrome, to name a few. Some babies are born to mothers who are addicted to drugs or alcohol, resulting in birth defects, and some suffer injuries such as shaken baby syndrome, burns, malnutrition, and broken bones, due to abuse or neglect. Still more children fall victim to childhood cancers, such as leukemia. Regardless of the injury, these children need help in order to develop in a normal manner and to be able to function within society to their utmost capabilities.

Many children are seen in specialty treatment centers, such as children's hospitals like St. Jude's Hospital or the Shriner's Burn Hospital. Occupational therapy intervention may include the facilitation of normal development patterns, neurodevelopmental training (NDT), splint fabrication, and range of motion (ROM). When possible, play activities are employed to meet these goals.

For school-age children (usually age five and up), occupational therapy can be conducted through their school districts. In 1975, Public Law PL 94-142, the Education for All Handicapped Children Act, made public school education available to all children, regardless of disability. In 1997, Public Law PL 105-17, the Individuals with Disabilities Education Act (IDEA), was established to provide for those students with special educational needs. In this setting, the occupational therapist attempts to help the child with the skills needed to participate in the educational process. These skills can include handwriting training, use of assistive technology, feeding, dressing, and toileting training.

Other Practice Areas

Although the vast majority of occupational therapists and occupational therapy assistants work in the traditional areas of mental health, physical dysfunction, and pediatrics, there are other, more uncommon practice areas to work in as well. An occupational therapist can work with any person who experiences a disruption of occupational roles. This opens up a wealth of prospective work environments for occupational therapists and occupational therapy assistants. These work arenas are typically referred to as "nontraditional" practice areas and include hospices, prisons, homeless shelters, and women's shelters.

Hospice and Palliative Care

Hospice work is near and dear to me, personally, because it is an area in which I have been involved for over 20 years. Hospice is a concept that began in England in the late 1960s to serve the needs of the terminally ill and their families. One might think (as I did at one time), "What good can occupational therapy do for terminally ill people? Aren't they just going to die?"

Believe it or not, working with the terminally ill taught me the true meaning of occupational therapy and its importance to the lives of anyone with an impairment of occupational roles. If I can make a difference in the life of a terminally ill client by allowing him to participate in the occupation of his choice—in essence, helping him to live until he dies— I can make a difference in anyone's life.

Prison

Although few occupational therapists actually work in the penal system, this is an area that can be greatly served by the profession. Prisons exist to punish those who have broken the laws of society, and there is certainly a need for the institution. Some people believe that we should "lock criminals up and throw away the key." However, many—if not most—prisoners are eventually released back into society. The question then becomes: "What do they do once they are free?" This is where occupational therapy can play an important role.

I pointed out in Chapter 1 that people who have too much time on their hands often get into trouble with the law and frequently end up in jail. This inability to utilize time effectively, combined with unemployment and substance abuse, can contribute to criminal behavior. If these individuals do not learn how to use their time effectively before being incarcerated, how can they be expected to utilize their time effectively after being released?

I pointed out in Chapter 2 that, in the past, many mentally ill individuals ended up in prison rather than receive the help they needed. Sadly, despite the Age of Enlightenment and the Reformation, the wheel of history continues to turn and repeat itself. Many of those currently incarcerated in the United States are mentally ill, and prison is not necessarily the treatment most beneficial to them. Many of these individuals were homeless prior to incarceration, and many will return to that lifestyle upon their release.

Those who are serving time in prison are also subject to the same illnesses and disabilities as those on the outside—possibly even more so. Prisoners who suffer strokes, cardiac, and orthopedic problems require rehabilitation for their injuries. Many in prison have HIV disease or full-blown AIDS. Many contract cancer and other terminal illnesses and may require palliative care in the final days of their lives.

While it is true that the purpose of prison is to punish, we cannot expect this punishment to instill upon them the skills necessary to resume life in a free society so that they do not, once again, break the law and return to prison. Occupational therapy can help to rehabilitate and, in some cases, habilitate them; to teach them the skills that are necessary to function within the boundaries of society; and to help them to cope with life on the outside.

Homeless Shelters

Within the United States of America, perhaps the greatest society in the history of humankind, there is a deep, dark, and yet, open secret: homelessness. We are all aware of the problem—we all see the bag lady, or the wino pushing his shopping cart down the street and sleeping in a cardboard box in any available alley—but we don't want to talk about it or acknowledge that it is a problem.

Many homeless people are mentally ill. Many of them are substance abusers. Many, however, are entire families who have been forced onto the streets by circumstances beyond their control (such as events like Hurricane Katrina). These people need help and guidance in order to get back on track. Homeless shelters can provide a safe place for those living on the streets, and occupational therapists can help homeless people reestablish themselves and find suitable work.

Women's Shelters

Another growing area for occupational therapists is in centers for victims of domestic violence. Women who come to these centers frequently have nowhere else to turn to escape an abusive partner. More often than not, these women have children, low self-esteem, and few, if any, skills required to function independently.

The occupational therapist working in this setting may focus on activities that promote self-esteem, child-care skills, time-management skills, and other areas that will help the client not only to function more independently, but also to develop the skills she will need to find and succeed at employment.

SUMMARY

This chapter has described the different employment settings where occupational therapists can be found. The traditional settings include psychiatric facilities, inpatient and outpatient settings, and home health.

Occupational therapy personnel can also be found in school systems. Due to the inclusive nature of school-based programs, occupational therapy is considered an important service for students.

Nontraditional settings, such as hospice programs, prisons, homeless shelters, and women's centers for victims of domestic abuse, were also discussed in this chapter.

CHAPTER 6

How Does Occupational Therapy Fit Into the Health Care Team?

Chapter Goals

At the conclusion of this chapter, the reader should understand the relationship between the occupational therapist and other members of the health care and educational team, including:

- the patient
- the family/significant others
- the physician
- nurses
- certified nurse aides
- physical therapists
- speech-language pathologists (speech therapists)
- therapeutic recreation and activities therapists

- dietitians

- vocational rehabilitation counselors

- teachers

Introduction

Having spent all of this time telling you how wonderful the profession of occupational therapy is, you must certainly be wondering how it fits in with the rest of the health care team and what these other professionals do. We will cover that subject matter in this chapter.

Occupational therapy—or any other health care profession, for that matter—cannot possibly address every aspect of the patient's life; the process requires teamwork. No member of the team is more or less important than any other member. Each team member has her own particular expertise to add to the overall solution (see Figure 6-1).

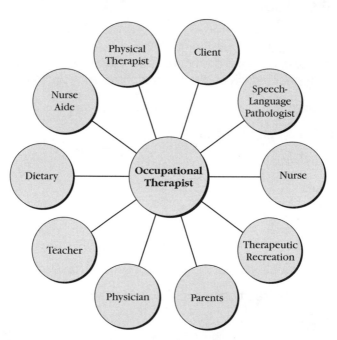

Figure 6-1. OT's relation to other professions

The Patient

I'll start with the patient because he is the most important, pivotal part of the team, and—more often than not—he is not even considered a part of the team. Frequently, the patient is acted upon by the team rather than treated as someone who interacts with the team.

Let's look at this from a slightly different perspective. Assume that you own a private advertising agency, and you have been hired to produce an ad campaign for which your client is to pay you $10 million. Great! You immediately go to work. You discuss the campaign with a copy-writer, a copy editor, a photographer, and a graphic artist. You select models, as well as the site for the photo shoot. You arrange the entire campaign and carry it out in magazines, television, and radio. The campaign runs for eight weeks, and then you realize that you forgot one thing: you never consulted with your client after the initial meeting. You call her up and take her to lunch. She is absolutely furious with you, because the campaign was nothing like she had envisioned it. She berates you for not consulting with her prior to its release. She tells you that not only will she never use your agency again, she will tell everyone she knows not to use you either. To add insult to injury, she tells you that you will be hearing from her attorney in the near future.

Of course, you would never do anything without consulting your client nearly every step of the way, would you? When it comes to health care, however, the client is usually the least informed or consulted member of the team, and most (if not all) decisions are made by the health care team with little or no input from the patient.

You must put yourself in the patient's place. Perhaps you've already been there. Your doctor or therapist tells you what they are going to do without asking you how you feel about it; you are not even included. How do you feel? You may feel angry, abandoned, and alone. How would you want to be treated? You would certainly want to have some input into the decisions that will affect your life. Why shouldn't everyone have that choice?

The Family/Significant Others

The family and significant others are also a very important part of the health care team. These are the people who spend the most time with the patient and who will be responsible, in part or in full, for carrying out the patient's health care program.

Like the patient, the family is often left out of the picture. Decisions may be made about the patient without being discussed beforehand with the family or significant others. These people are often confused by medical jargon, or "medicalese," which they are unable to understand. Many people are also intimidated by medical personnel and will rarely ask questions.

On the other hand, sometimes the family and medical staff form a secret pact in which both sides are in regular, open communication while the patient is excluded from the details of his condition. This is especially true in the case of serious or terminal illness. Everyone may believe that it is in the patient's best interest to be kept in the dark about his prognosis. This is not only unfair, it is also unethical. All patients have the right to know their diagnosis and prognosis; this is known as **diagnostic honesty** in **hospice** care. Unfortunately, this is rarely practiced, and the legacy of secrecy continues on a daily basis.

The Physician

There was a time when the doctor was *the* most important person on the health care team; these days, the physician—although still very important— has become more of a manager who delegates responsibilities to other members. The physician is responsible for the overall treatment plan, which is usually accomplished through referrals and by writing prescriptions for specific services, including occupational therapy.

In the modern reality of managed care, most people have a **primary care physician** (PCP) to whom they turn with general medical problems; in the good old days, this person was known as the family doctor. The PCP typically diagnoses and treats the run-of-the-mill disorders that one acquires on a regular basis, and serves as a **gatekeeper** for any additional, specialized medical services, such as **neurology, physiatry, gastroenterology, psychiatry,** and so on.

Any physician can order occupational therapy for a given patient; however, most orders for occupational therapy come from the PCP, **internists,** physiatrists, neurologists, and (far less frequently) psychiatrists.

Regardless of which physician orders occupational therapy, the therapist has a responsibility to respond to, and follow, those orders as written. For example, the physician may write an order specifying "OT eval and treat as necessary." The occupational therapist must then evaluate the patient (usually within 48 hours of receipt of the order) and determine the treatment plan. Occasionally, the results of the evaluation reveal no need for further therapy, and the patient is discharged. Typically, however, the therapist completes the evaluation, formulates a treatment plan, and implements treatment.

Communication with the physician is performed regularly via several methods: in person, by telephone, and in writing. The initial occupational therapy treatment plan must be signed by the physician before it is considered valid. Regular updates on the patient's progress are sent to the physician at specified intervals or as the patient's condition warrants.

Regular communication with the physician is imperative, and most of this communication is written. Regardless of how the communication occurs, it must be documented and entered into the patient's chart for legal and reimbursement reasons.

Nurses

The nurse is the heart, soul, and backbone of the medical profession; without nurses, the health care field would be in total disarray. The occupational therapist will inevitably have regular, frequent interactions with nursing personnel.

Nurses are trained to help their patients and, essentially, to do things for them—not to let them do things for themselves. Sometimes this philosophy can put the nurse at odds with the occupational therapist, whose job it is to make the client do things for himself. As you might guess, these opposite approaches to care may lead to some problems.

Once again, good communication between the occupational therapist and the nursing staff is extremely important. While the therapist must respect the wishes and efforts of the nurse, who is primarily concerned with the health and safety of the patient, she must also impress upon the nursing staff the importance of allowing the patient to do things for himself.

Certified Nurse Aides

If the nurse is the backbone of the health care profession, then the certified nurse aide (CNA) is most certainly the muscles. The certified nurse aide probably has more direct contact with the patient than any other medical professional. The certified nurse aide helps patients with most activities of daily living (ADLs), such as bathing, dressing, grooming, and toileting. He also frequently helps the patients eat meals and transports them from one place to another.

Because certified nurse aides work so closely with the patient, they inevitably become associated with occupational therapy, at least in terms of ADL training. Occupational therapists can, and often do, work closely with certified nurse aides in this regard.

Like the nurse, the nurse aide's job is to do things for the patient. Nurse aids are the workhorses of the medical profession and, sadly, are often the least respected and lowest-paid members of the medical team. The nurse aide probably spends more time with patients than any other member of the team, bathing, dressing, transferring, and feeding them. They are also the ones who are called upon to clean the patient, in the event of an episode of bowel or bladder **incontinence.** In short, the nurse aide does most of the dirty work and gets little recognition.

To add insult to injury, nurse aides are notoriously overworked and short staffed. This often results in anger and resentment on the part of the nurse aide, who may vent her frustration on the patient. The relationship between the nurse aide and the occupational therapist can here play a vital role in patient care.

The occupational therapist can **screen** potential patients for therapy by consulting with the nurse aide. The therapist can then **evaluate** the patient, determine the problem areas, and work on those problems. By helping the patient to do things such as bathing, dressing, and self-feeding, the occupational therapist not only helps the patient but lightens the load of the nurse aide, as well: a win-win situation for everyone involved!

Physical Therapists

Physical therapists (PTs) and physical therapy assistants (PTAs) are concerned with helping people to gain or regain the use of muscles and strengthen weakened muscles. The physical therapist uses exercise to achieve these goals, including isometric, isotonic, and resistive exercise using weights or elastic bands. Physical therapists also use modalities such as heat packs, contrast baths, ultrasounds, and electrical stimulation to relieve pain and facilitate movement and strength.

The focus of physical therapy, in many instances, is to increase an individual's ability to walk. As a person's strength increases, he is (hopefully) able to go from a wheelchair to a walker, then to a cane, and eventually to independent ambulation.

Occupational therapists work very closely with physical therapists, perhaps more than any other health professionals. There are many overlaps in the education and treatment approaches of both professions, and they are frequently confused by the general public. Not a week goes by without someone asking me "What's the difference between occupational therapy and physical therapy?" My answer is always the same: "about five dollars an hour." Seriously, despite the role confusion and frequent professional jealousy, the two professions are unique and have much to offer those who need their services.

Speech-Language Pathologists (Speech Therapists)

Speech therapists do more than just help people to speak properly, despite their job title. Speech-language pathologists are very involved with cognitive retraining (as are occupational therapists) and swallowing problems, or **dysphagia.**

All human functions, both automatic and voluntary, begin in the brain. Speech, perhaps the highest of all cognitive abilities, is a complex phenomenon that involves both expressive and receptive components, as well as short- and long-term memory. When there is a problem involving the parts of the brain responsible for speech, there can be a subsequent problem expressing or understanding language.

Some occupational therapists also work with swallowing disorders; however, I personally believe that this is a highly specialized area of practice that should not be attempted by a novice, due to the invasive nature of the activity and the inherent dangers, including choking and inhaling food, which may lead to pneumonia and death. Therefore, anyone who attempts this aspect of treatment must receive specialized training.

Therapeutic Recreation and Activities Therapists

Although occupational therapy and therapeutic recreation both sprang from the same historic roots, and sometimes seem to be very similar, major differences exist between the two professions. While occupational therapy focuses on work, self-care, and play and leisure, a great deal of emphasis has not been applied to the play and leisure aspect in recent years. With the exception of children's play, occupational therapists have primarily passed that area of focus on to recreational therapists. One major difference between the two professions, however, is salary.

An activities therapist is actually a recreational therapist; however, a recreational therapist has typically earned a bachelor's degree, along with certification from the National Council for Therapeutic Recreation Certification (NCTRC). Activities therapy is designed to keep people busily involved in activities that may or may not have a therapeutic goal, other than simply being fun. A certified occupational therapy assistant (COTA) can function as an activities therapist and does not require occupational therapist, registered (OTR) supervision in this role.

Dietitians

The relationship between occupational therapy and diet is a limited one, but it can be very important.

Each patient has different dietary needs. Diabetics must avoid too much sugar, while people with high blood pressure must avoid salt or sodium in their diets. The foods that we eat play a vital role in our health. Occupational therapists must be aware of the special dietary needs of their patients and encourage them to adhere to any necessary requirements.

The occupational therapist's job is to make sure that the patient can feed himself as much as possible; it doesn't do any good for a patient to have a special diet if he cannot eat the food. The occupational therapist consults with dietitians concerning the physical needs of the patient, primarily involving the process of getting food from the plate to his mouth in the easiest and most efficient manner possible.

The occupational therapist first evaluates the individual's strengths and weaknesses in terms of physical and mental abilities. The therapist utilizes an arsenal of assistive devices to aid the feeding process, beginning with something as simple as noting how the client is positioned during a meal, or making the handle of his fork bigger and easier to hold, to providing him with a lipped plate to prevent food from sliding off. In the case of a severely disabled individual, the occupational therapist may recommend and order a high-tech feeding device that can be controlled by the client using a head pointer or other adaptation.

The consistency of the food will often make a difference in a person's ability to eat. Someone with no teeth, for example, would find it difficult to eat a piece of uncut steak, and, therefore, the steak needs to be cut up for her. Alternatively, the occupational therapist could teach the client how to easily cut her own steak using assistive devices such as a **rocker knife** or a pizza wheel.

People with conditions such as **Parkinson's disease** often have difficulty swallowing their food. This can cause choking or the inhaling (**aspiration**) of food, which can lead to pneumonia. The occupational therapist, often in tandem with the speech-language pathologist and dietitian, can assist these individuals by thickening their food and beverages to prevent choking.

Vocational Rehabilitation Counselors

The rehabilitation counselor's job entails helping individuals with disabilities to find employment. Many of these individuals have physical or emotional problems that prevent them from participating in gainful employment. Rehabilational counselors "provide personal and vocational counseling, and arrange for medical care, vocational training and job placement" (www.stats.bls.gov/oco/ocos067.htm, 6/26/05). The rehabilitation counselor often consults with an occupational therapist to assist individuals in overcoming their disabilities enough to maintain employment.

Many rehabilitation counselors are employed in state positions, such as each state's Office of Vocational Rehabilitation. Many of their clients have conditions such as **cerebral palsy, mental retardation, blindness,** and **traumatic brain injuries.** Many other clients may have job-acquired injuries and might receive **workers' compensation** or other disability compensation. Whatever the cause of the disability, the occupational therapist can contribute significant input that will help place the client in an appropriate employment situation.

Teachers

The teacher is not part of the health care team but is the central member of the educational team. In these days of inclusion, more and more students with physical, emotional, and learning disabilities are being admitted to public schools and require special attention from many professionals, including occupational therapists.

The Individuals with Disabilities Education Act (IDEA) requires that all public school children who receive special education must have an **Individualized Education Program** (IEP), which is specially designed for each individual student. The teacher and all other participating professionals, including occupational therapists, must provide input for the IEP that essentially comprises a special education treatment plan.

A child's primary occupational role in the school setting is that of student. In this setting, the occupational therapist focuses on problem areas that interfere with the student role. Some common problems addressed by the school-based occupational therapist include handwriting, positioning, attention-deficit hyperactivity disorder (ADHD), and developmental disabilities such as mental retardation, cerebral palsy, muscular dystrophy, and cystic fibrosis, among others.

Activities of daily living, such as toileting, dressing, and self-feeding skills, may also be addressed in the school system, as these are necessary skills for students attending school.

Summary

This chapter has described the role of the occupational therapist and occupational therapy assistant as part of either a health care or educational team. The relationship between occupational therapists and the various professionals with whom they work closely has been described. A thumbnail sketch of these professions has also been presented.

The salient concept of this chapter is that the client or patient, as well as his family and significant others, is the centerpiece and most important member of the team and should always have a central role in the direction of his plan of care.

CHAPTER 7

The Occupational Therapy Process

Chapter Goals

At the conclusion of this chapter, the reader should:

- Have a basic understanding of some of the commonly used terminology in the profession of occupational therapy.
- Know how occupational therapy referrals are generated.
- Know the difference between a screening and an evaluation.
- Know the various components of the occupational therapy evaluation process.
- Understand the basic components of the treatment process.
- Know when and why a client is discharged from occupational therapy services.

INTRODUCTION

This chapter is intended to familiarize you, the reader, with some of the common terminology used in the profession of occupational therapy. In a way, it is a glossary of terms. I have presented this information in narrative form, in order to put the definitions into a context that is easier to understand.

The chapter will begin at the referral level and then proceed through the evaluation, treatment, and discharge levels. This is a general overview, and, due to the diverse areas of practice, I have taken a bit of artistic license (although I have been told many times that I should have my artistic license revoked) by combining physical disabilities, pediatrics, psychiatry, and other areas in order to reduce confusion and maintain the flow of the material. I hope that you will find the material a bit easier to understand.

The Occupational Therapy Referral and Evaluation

Before occupational therapy intervention can occur, the therapist must receive a **referral** for services. This referral typically comes from a physician and is frequently accompanied by a prescription for treatment. This prescription may be as specific as fabricating a splint for an injured hand or as general as "occupational therapy to evaluate and treat." If the therapist intends to be reimbursed by a **third party payer**—such as Medicare, Medicaid, Blue Cross/Blue Shield, and so forth—for services rendered, she must receive a physician's referral. If the client approaches the therapist and agrees to pay for services out of pocket (known as **private pay**), a referral is not necessary. It should be noted that private pay occupational therapy occurs rarely.

Another exception to the physician referral is the school-based referral for occupational therapy. Occupational therapists are an important part of the education team and frequently work with students in the school system. Virtually anyone who is involved with the student—from parents to teachers—can request an occupational therapy assessment.

Some therapists may attempt to increase their **caseloads** (the number of clients that they treat) by performing occupational therapy **screenings.** A screening is when the therapist meets with a client and performs a cursory evaluation of that individual's occupational needs. If the therapist determines that the client would benefit from occupational therapy services, he can request a referral from that person's primary physician. The occupational therapy screening is typically a *gratis* service; that is, third party payers will not reimburse for this service. However, this is an important service because the screening can identify those who may need occupational therapy services but would have slipped through the cracks otherwise.

The Evaluation Process

Once the referral is received, the therapist can perform an **initial evaluation** of the client. This evaluation assesses physical, cognitive, and developmental functioning, and how any impairments are impacting the client's occupational role performance. The evaluation is the foundation upon which the occupational therapy treatment plan is built.

The Initial Interview and Occupational History

Upon meeting for the first time, the occupational therapist introduces herself to the client (and the family, if any are present) and begins by explaining exactly what occupational therapy is and how it can help to make the client more independent in the areas of self-care, work, and play and leisure. This first meeting is extremely important, because it sets the stage for the entire relationship between the client and the therapist, as well as forming the client's perception of occupational therapy in general. The old adage "you never get a second chance to make a first impression" rings true in this situation.

At this time, the therapist administers an **occupational history** (Figure 7–1) to the client and, if appropriate, to the client's caregiver. The occupational history, first described by Linda Moorhead (1969), is a series of probing questions (according to Brinkman and Kirschner, "Friends pry, medical professionals probe") that helps the therapist obtain information about the client that can be used to facilitate the therapeutic relationship and, ultimately, develop a seamless treatment plan. Unlike so many other professional interview methods, the occupational history is designed to assess the client "as a person first, and as a medical condition, second" (Tigges and Marcil, 1988, p. 119).

The occupational history helps the therapist learn about the client's work history, including education, training (it includes a section for paid employment as well as for homemakers), and personal and family history, including where the client grew up, what her interests are, and what she enjoys doing. Finally, it includes questions about how the client spends her time—both before and since her illness or injury. Ultimately, the occupational history asks three salient questions upon which the occupational therapist can base her treatment plan:

- What are the most important things that your illness or injury has prevented you from doing?
- At the present time, what brings you the greatest pleasure?
- What are the things that you would most like to do right now?

A. Work History (Employment)

1. I understand that before you became ill/injured, you were a
   _____. What an interesting job! How did you become interested
   in that line of work?
2. What sort of training/education was involved?
3. Where did you get your training?
4. What was the first job you had?
5. What jobs did you have after that?
6. What was the last job you had before you became ill/injured?
7. What did your job actually entail?
8. Did you work up until you became ill/injured?
9. (If retired) How long have you been retired?

B. Work History (Homemaker)

1. I understand that you have been a homemaker/parent for many
   years. That is more than a full-time job, isn't it?
2. What is the most challenging thing about being a homemaker? A
   spouse? A parent?
3. What is the most frustrating part about being a homemaker? A
   spouse? A parent?
4. Are you involved in community activities? If yes, what are they?
5. Were you still active in these until you became ill/injured?
6. Since you became ill/injured, what things have been most difficult to
   give up?
7. What bothers you the most about the things you've had to give up?
8. What type of work is/was your spouse involved with?

C. Family History

1. Have you always lived in (city/state)? If not, where did you live
   before you moved here?
2. What do/did your parents do for a living?
3. Do you have any brothers or sisters? Where do they live? Do you see
   or talk to them often?
4. I understand that you have children/grandchildren. Where do they
   live? Do you see or talk to them frequently?
5. Before you became ill/injured, what were your duties/responsibilities
   around the house?
6. Before you became ill/injured, what did you do for fun and
   relaxation?
7. What are the most important things that your illness/injury has
   prevented you from doing?
8. At the present time, what brings you the greatest pleasure?
9. What are the things that you would most like to do now?

Figure 7-1. The occupational history helps the therapist to see
the patient as a person first and a diagnosis second.

These three questions can provide the occupational therapist with the most important information for developing an effective treatment plan. The talented occupational therapist or occupational therapy assistant can take these individual pieces of the client's life, combine them with the physical findings of the evaluation, and use them to enhance the treatment process.

The Temporal Assessment

Also important in the development of the treatment plan is finding out how the client uses time or, conversely, is used by time. Most of us have a daily schedule or routine to which we adhere. We typically get up at the same time each day and go to bed around the same time each night. In between, we usually have an idea of what needs to be done each day. This schedule may differ on weekends, but, even then, we tend to have a schedule for those days as well.

When one becomes ill or injured, one's daily schedule is completely disrupted, and a person may find himself languishing in bed all day, occasionally dozing off, and waking to eat or watch television. Eventually, one loses all track of time and ultimately loses the desire to participate in life's activities.

The occupational therapist needs to have an idea of what the client's schedule was like before she became ill or injured. A **Temporal Adaptation Assessment** (Figure 7–2) may be administered in order to get an idea of how the client uses time (the word *temporal* is a fancy way of saying time). While most people are able to adhere to a schedule of some sort, there are many people do not use time well, which may result in problems such as chronic lateness, missing things like a bus, a plane, or a class, and procrastination. The inability to use time well can also result in constant anxiety, because the person feels helpless to accomplish tasks in a timely and effective manner.

The occupational therapist will often administer an **interest inventory** to supplement the occupational history. The interest inventory, first described by Janice Matsutsuyu (1969), is a list of various activities and games that the client checks off as appropriate. This information can also help the therapist choose activities for the client during therapy.

Caring for the Caregiver

Sometimes it is also necessary to interview the caregiver in order to determine her own needs (Marcil and Tigges, 1992). In many cases, the client may be totally dependent for all of his care, as, for example, in the cases of advanced Alzheimer's disease, end-stage cancer, or end-stage Tay-Sachs

1. Before you became ill/injured, was it important for you to have a daily schedule? In what ways was it important or not important to you?

2. How did you organize a typical day? Start from the time you got up in the morning and include everything you did until you went to bed.

3. What is your daily schedule like now?

4. If you had your choice, how would you like to spend tomorrow?

Figure 7-2. The Temporal Adaptation Assessment helps the therapist determine how the patient uses time or is used by time.

disease. In cases such as these, there is often little that the occupational therapist can legitimately do for the client. However, the caregiver can frequently benefit from recommendations made by the occupational therapist. When the client is a child, the caregiver can frequently be provided helpful hints for caring for the child and following through with the therapy program.

The caregiver frequently gets lost in the shuffle and has no personal time. Many caregivers are in a position of caring for their aging parents as well as their young children, all of whom need their time and attention. This so-called "sandwich generation" is under a great deal of stress due to these constant demands. If we factor in part-time or full-time employment, the stress level can become astronomical; this is a real dilemma for thousands of people on a daily basis. If this scenario is left unresolved, it can lead to caregiver anger and resentment, depression, and hopelessness. It is not uncommon to read in the newspaper about a caregiver who snapped and committed suicide after murdering her charge. It is extremely important to attend to, and care for, the caregiver as well as the client. This care and attention can start with a few simple questions (Figure 7–3).

Muscle and Joint Assessment

The functional evaluation typically begins with an assessment of the client's physical functioning. The occupational therapist tends to focus on the upper extremities more than the lower ones. The individual's **range of motion** (ROM)—the extent to which a joint can move—is tested to see if he can move his arms and fingers, or if there are any impairments of movement. Joint movement is measured using a device called a **goniometer** (*gonio* = angle, *meter* = to measure), which measures joint movement from 0° to 180° (Figure 7–4).

1. How are you managing with the physical care of (the client)?

2. What are the things that you are having the most difficulty doing for (the client)?

3. What would you like help with in caring for (the client)?

4. How are you coping with your personal life? Do you get a chance to get out and do important things for yourself?

Figure 7-3. The Caregiver Assessment determines how the caregiver is coping with the caregiver role.

There are two kinds of range of motion: passive and active. **Passive range of motion** (PROM) is the amount of joint movement available when the therapist moves the joint, and the client is relaxed and merely goes along for the ride. **Active range of motion** (AROM) is the amount of joint movement available from the client, of his own muscle power and volition, with no help from the therapist. When the client is given a little bit of help from the therapist, **active assisted range of motion** (AAROM) occurs. Most of us have greater PROM than AROM, because most people stop a movement when they experience tightness or pain. Therapists can achieve greater passive range from clients, because they don't care about the client's pain and discomfort (that's not really true). Actually, a seasoned therapist can bring a joint to maximal PROM and knows when to stop before hurting the client. Figure 7–5 provides a list of the normal ranges of motion for all joints in the human body.

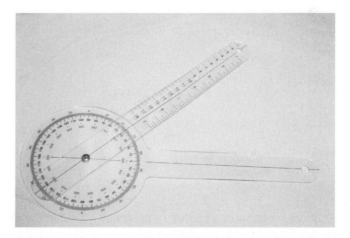

Figure 7-4. The goniometer is a device that can accurately measure the range of motion in joints.

Cervical Spine

Flexion	0–45
Extension	0–45
Lateral flexion	0–45
Rotation	0–60

Thoracic and Lumbar Spine

Flexion	0–170
Extension	0–60
Lateral flexion	0–40
Rotation	0–45

Shoulder

Flexion	0–170
Extension	0–60
Abduction	0–170
Horizontal abduction	0–40
Horizontal adduction	0–130
Internal rotation	0–70
External rotation	0–90

Elbow and Forearm

Flexion	0–145
Extension	0
Supination	0–85
Pronation	0–85

Wrist

Flexion	0–80
Extension	0–70
Ulnar deviation	0–30
Radial deviation	0–20

Thumb

MP flexion	0–50
IP flexion	0–85
Abduction	0–50

Fingers

MP flexion	0–50
MP extension	0–40
PIP flexion	0–110
DIP flexion	0–80
Abduction	0–25

Hip

Flexion	0–120
Extension	0–30

Figure 7-5. The range of normal joint motion, as measured by a goniometer.

	Abduction	0–40
	Adduction	0–35
	Internal rotation	0–45
	External rotation	0–45
Knee		
	Flexion	0–135
Ankle and Foot		
	Plantar flexion	0–50
	Dorsiflexion	0–15
	Inversion	0–35
	Eversion	0–20

Figure 7-5. (Continued)

Next, and closely associated with ROM, is the testing of muscle strength. Weak muscles can interfere with AROM and impair daily activities. Muscle strength is tested in two ways: by a Manual Muscle Test and a dynamometer. When using the **Manual Muscle Test** (MMT), the therapist has the client attempt to move the muscle(s) in either a gravity-eliminated position (for weak muscles) or an anti-gravity position, with or without added resistance. An example of gravity-eliminated muscle testing would be to have the client position his elbow on a tabletop (to remove the force of gravity) and have him bend (or flex) his elbow. Testing this same muscle in an anti-gravity position would involve having the client hold his arm at his side and then bend his elbow; this causes the muscles to flex the elbow against the force of gravity. The results of this test allow the therapist to assign a letter or number grade, ranging from zero (no movement) to five (normal strength). Figure 7–6 provides the MMT scale.

The second method used to test muscle strength is a **dynamometer** (*dyn* = force, *meter* = measure); this is a device that is calibrated, or adjusted, to test the amount of force exerted by a single muscle or a group of muscles. Although a dynamometer can be used on any muscle group, occupational therapists typically use MMTs on all muscle groups except the hand. The dynamometer provides an objective measurement of hand-grip strength, and a **finger dynamometer** is used to specifically measure the pinch strength of the fingers. Figures 7–7a and 7–7b show a standard dynamometer and pinch dynamometer.

While performing ROM and MMT, the occupational therapist can also identify whether the patient has normal, little, or no muscle tone, known as **flaccidity,** or too much muscle tone, known as **spasticity.** Either of these conditions will impair an individual's ability to function adequately in daily activities.

5	Normal	N	The body part moves through full range of motion against maximum resistance and gravity.
	Good	G	The body part moves through full range of motion against gravity and moderate resistance.
	Fair plus	F+	The body part moves through full range of motion against gravity and minimal resistance.
3	Fair	F	The body part moves through full range of motion with no added resistance.
	Fair minus	F–	The body part moves through less-than-full range of motion against gravity.
	Poor plus	P+	The body part moves through full range of motion with gravity eliminated and then relaxes suddenly.
2	Poor	P	The body part moves through full range of motion with gravity eliminated and with no added resistance.
	Poor minus	P–	The body part moves through less-than-full range of motion with gravity eliminated.
1	Trace	T	Tension can be felt in the muscle but no movement occurs.
0	Zero	0	No muscle tension can be detected.

Adapted from Trombly, C. A. (1995). *Occupational therapy for physical dysfunction* (4th ed.). Baltimore, MD: Williams & Wilkins.

Figure 7-6. The Manual Muscle Test (MMT) is the most common method used by therapists to evaluate muscle strength.

Gross and Fine Motor Assessment

Occupational therapists tend to focus on the arms and hands during evaluation and treatment. This is primarily due to the fact that we use our arms and hands to do many things; therefore, how well they work has an impact on an individual's daily functioning.

Gross motor function refers to the large muscles or groups of muscles of the body. The word *gross* means large, and has nothing to do with what the exposed muscle looks like (as in "eeew, that's gross!"). Gross motor movement is usually made evident while active range of motion is being assessed. A simple example of gross motor movement would be waving your arms in the air.

Fine motor skills pertain to the smaller muscles found in the hands and the amount of dexterity an individual possesses. The ability to oppose ones fingers, to spread them and bring them back together, and to pick up and manipulate objects is important to perform activities such as writing, tying shoes, playing video games, text messaging, and using a cellular telephone.

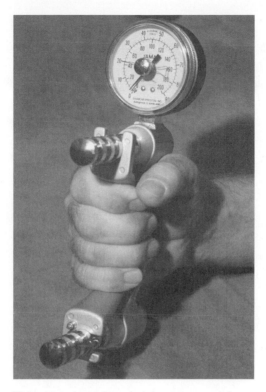

Figure 7-7a. The standard hand dynamometer is used to determine hand-grip strength.

Sensory Testing

The next step in the evaluation process is testing the client's sensation. You may recall that we have five basic senses: vision, hearing, smell, taste, and touch. These senses are important because they help us to effectively interact with, and survive within, our environment. If there is a malfunction of one or more of these senses, the client may have difficulty adapting to, and functioning with, a disability. The senses of vision, hearing, smell, and taste are fairly straightforward and do not require a great deal of explanation; the sense of touch, however, is a bit more complicated than most people realize, and occupational therapists frequently focus on this area.

We depend on our sense of touch without even thinking about it. When we touch an extremely hot or cold object, we pull away and protect ourselves. When we reach into a pocket or a purse and pull out a coin or another object without looking at it, we rely on our sense of touch to help us. Impairment of sensation can seriously impair function, particularly

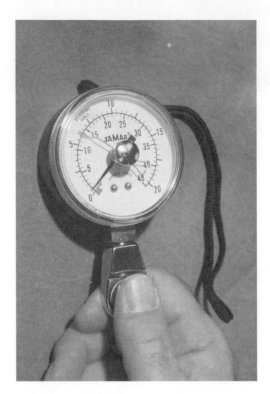

Figure 7-7b. The finger/pinch dynamometer is used to determine three types of pinch strength: two-point pinch, three-point pinch, and lateral (or key grip) pinch.

with respect to the hand. A hand without sensation is of little use, even if all motor functions and musculoskeletal structures are intact.

Have either one of your hands ever "fallen asleep"? It happens to most people every now and then. Personally, I hate it when my hand falls asleep during the day, because I know it will be up all night. Seriously, this condition, known as **neuropraxia,** occurs when a nerve has been pressed on for a short period of time. The result is numbness, tingling, and sometimes pain. We usually move our hand to "get the circulation going again" (although this is a fallacy about blood circulation). At any rate, that is what it feels like to lose sensation. A person may lose all sensation and feel absolutely nothing; this is called anesthesia (some people think that anesthesia is a Disney movie, but that is incorrect).

Let us look at the different aspects of this sensation, which occupational therapists frequently evaluate. Prior to testing sensation, the client is blindfolded or has his vision occluded in some other manner in order

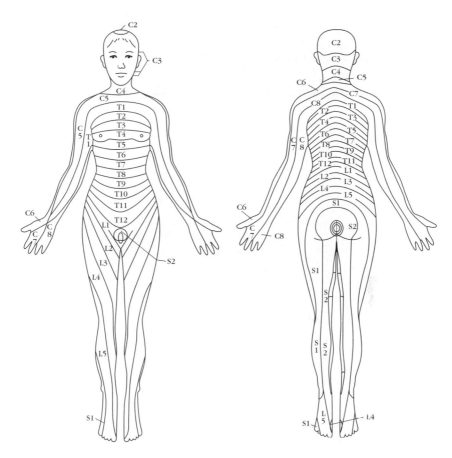

Figure 7-8. The dermatomes serve as a type of road map to determine which areas of the body are given sensation by which spinal nerves. The letter and number designations indicate the spinal level and the exact spinal nerve responsible for innervating a specific part of the body.

to prevent him from seeing what is being done, thereby prompting him to give the "right" answer. All sensory testing is performed in an orderly manner using the body's **dermatomes** (Greek for "skin cutting"). Dermatomes are areas of the body that are serviced by specific sensory nerves and essentially serve as a road map of the body to allow the therapist to determine what nerves may be impaired. Each area of the body is innervated by a specific peripheral nerve that exits the spinal cord at a specific place, identified by the vertebra from which it exits. There are eight cervical nerves, identified as C1, C2, C3, C4, C5, C6, C7, and C8.

Similarly, there are 12 thoracic nerves, identified as T1–T12; 5 lumbar nerves, identified as L1–L5; and 1 sacral nerve, S1. Each dermatome is identified by the spinal nerve that innervates it. Figure 7–8 shows the dermatome pattern of the human body.

Some of the **tactile** (related to the sense of touch) areas tested include **light touch** and **deep pressure,** the ability to detect two simultaneous touch stimuli at varied intervals (**two-point discrimination**), **thermal sensations** (hot and cold), and **superficial pain.** The ability to identify objects by feeling them without looking at them, known as **stereognosis,** is also tested, as well as the ability to identify the static position of a body part in space, known as **proprioception,** and the active movement of a body part through space, known as **kinesthetic awareness.**

Although stereognosis, kinesthesia, and proprioception are forms of sensation, they are considered higher forms that are determined by the brain's interpretation; therefore, they typically fall under the category of perception.

Cognitive and Perceptual Testing

When working with certain clients, such as those who have had a stroke, head injury, or other neurological impairment (such as cerebral palsy and Alzheimer's disease), the occupational therapist needs to assess the client's cognitive and perceptual abilities. People with mental illnesses may also have difficulty with the areas of cognition and perception, so they, too, are tested for these abilities.

Cognition is the mental process characterized by knowing, thinking, learning, understanding, and judging (*Mosby's Medical, Nursing, and Allied Health Dictionary*, 1998, 361). **Perception** is the conscious recognition and interpretation of sensory stimuli that serve as a basis for understanding, learning, and knowing (*Mosby's Medical, Nursing, and Allied Health Dictionary*, 1998, 1233).

Assessing cognitive impairments is a complex process and takes finely honed skills to perform well. The cognitive functions frequently assessed by the occupational therapist include attention, memory, initiation, planning and organization, mental flexibility, abstraction, insight, reasoning, problem solving, and judgment (Wheatley, 2001). Again, these areas are also important when working with the mentally ill.

A person with an impairment of one or more components of cognition may not only be unable to carry out activities of daily living, he may also be a danger to himself or others. For example, a woman with Alzheimer's disease may have difficulty remembering things or planning and initiating an activity. If this woman lives alone and attempts to cook herself dinner, she might light the stove, put food on the burner, and then leave the room, completely forgetting about her task; this could lead to a catastrophic house fire. Therefore, the occupational therapist must have a strong understanding of the client's cognitive abilities before designing a treatment plan.

All too often, we hear stories about people—usually elderly—who have wandered away from their homes, only to be hit by a car or found dead due to drowning, exposure, or a similar cause. Many elderly people die in house fires that probably could have been prevented if they had been identified as mentally at-risk persons.

Assessment of perceptual abilities are equally complex and require focused training on the part of the occupational therapist. Perception refers to the way in which the brain interprets sensory input and involves all senses. Perception is reality, and, depending on how one perceives a given stimulus, what one perceives is what one believes—even if one's perception is wrong.

For example, when I was a teenager, I was a member of a club with limited membership. New members were initiated into our club by participating in a ritual that went like this: The inductee was instructed to remove his shoes and socks. He was then blindfolded. A glass bottle was broken nearby, and the inductee was ordered to walk forward. If he resisted, he was pushed forward, which usually resulted in bloodcurdling screams as his bare feet landed squarely on the cornflakes that had been secretly sprinkled on the ground in front of him. He, of course, perceived that he was stepping on broken glass, because that is what his senses (incorrectly) told him.

When a client experiences a stroke, or other neurological insults, the brain may frequently misinterpret the information that the senses provide. This misinterpretation can make life difficult or even dangerous. For example, a stroke survivor may develop a **left-sided neglect,** wherein he does not see or pay attention to things in his left visual field, without even realizing that he cannot see these things. This inability to attend to his left side could cause him to bump into doorways, furniture, and other items, resulting in falls or injuries.

Another common result of left-sided neglect is evident during meals. Individuals will eat all of the food on the right side of the plate and not even realize that there is still food remaining on the other side. If you were to observe these individuals eat, you would think that they had taken a knife and divided the plate into two equal halves, leaving all of the food on the left half untouched!

Similarly, someone who has had a limb—such as an arm or a leg—amputated will often say that he has an itch on his foot or a pain in his big toe, even though the foot is no longer there; this is a phenomenon known as **phantom limb sensation** or, in the case of pain, **phantom pain sensation.** Even though the body part is no longer actually there, the remaining nerve endings tell the brain that it is. Consequently, it still feels to the person as though the limb exists. The sensation of the limb and the experience of the pain are real.

Other areas of perception frequently addressed by the occupational therapist include: stereognosis, graphesthesia, body scheme, and praxis. **Stereognosis,** discussed earlier in this chapter, is the ability to identify objects through feel, without looking at them. A similar perceptual test exists for **graphesthesia,** the ability to identify letters and numbers traced on the skin. If you were to close your eyes and have someone trace letters on the palm of your hand, you should be able to correctly interpret and identify those letters.

Occupational therapists often test their client's ability to plan and perform purposeful movements; this is known as **praxis.** The impairment of praxis is called **apraxia,** which is defined as "the execution of learned movement which cannot be accounted for by either weakness, incoordination, or sensory loss, or by incomprehension of or inattention to commands" (Geschwind, 1975, 168). This condition can impair one's ability to perform simple activities such as dressing and writing, among many others.

Body scheme is the way in which an individual perceives her own body. Most of us think of our body as if we were looking at a recent photograph of ourselves. Following a neurological insult or psychiatric condition, a person's body scheme can change dramatically. After a stroke, a man might not realize that his affected arm actually belongs to him, and he may pick it up and attempt to throw it away. A 90-pound girl with anorexia nervosa, a serious eating disorder, may perceive herself as morbidly obese and, therefore, stop eating in order to lose weight.

Assessing Activities of Daily Living

Activities of daily living (ADLs) are the common things that we perform on a regular or quasi-regular basis. These include, but are not limited to, activities such as dressing, toileting, writing, and using a telephone. ADLs are generally considered to be the basic tasks that one performs. Higher-level, more complex tasks are referred to as **instrumental activities of daily living** (IADLs); for example, while self-feeding is considered an ADL, preparing a meal is an IADL. Dressing is an ADL, while washing, ironing, and folding clothes are a more complex series of tasks considered to be IADLs. The occupational therapist has a duty to assess a client's ability to perform ADLs and IADLs, and to help her perform those activities that are important to her. The best way to assess these skills is by actually having the client perform them to the best of her ability while the therapist observes. Therefore, the occupational therapist evaluates the client while she performs such activities as dressing, bathing, grooming, transferring, and toileting. Other activities, such as meal planning and preparation, homemaking, and driving skills, are also evaluated.

Once these skills have been assessed, the occupational therapist can determine which areas are in need of improvement and, after consulting with the client and his significant others, begin to develop a **treatment plan** for that individual. This consultation is extremely important;if the client does not want to work on the goals that the therapist has deemed important, that client may not be very cooperative, and the goal(s) may never be achieved.

Treatment Planning

Once all of the important data is gathered, the occupational therapist puts it together in a comprehensive treatment plan. The treatment plan is based on two things: 1) the client's needs, and 2) the client's interests and desires. The treatment plan lays out objectives that the client is expected to meet through active participation in therapy. These objectives are typically divided into **short-term goals** and **long-term goals.**

A short-term goal is one that can be achieved in a relatively short time frame—that is, within a day, a week, a month, and so forth. The short-term goal also significantly contributes to the achievement of the broader long-term goal.

A long-term goal is the ultimate objective toward which the therapist and the client are striving. For example, a long-term goal for Mrs. Mendoza is for her to independently don her bra and blouse. The steps needed to reach that long term goal are the short-term goals. In this case, her short-term goals may include increasing the strength in her arms and shoulders, increasing the active range of motion in her arms and shoulders to within normal limits (WNL), and improving the fine motor dexterity in both hands to allow her to manipulate buttons and clasps.

As Figure 7–9 depicts, short-term goals are like steps leading up to the top of the staircase, where the long-term goal is waiting patiently.

A good goal should be a S.M.A.R.T. goal: Specific, Measurable, Attainable, Realistic, and Timely.

"Specific" indicates exactly what the goal intends to do. For example, instead of saying that "Mr. Jones will get stronger" (not specific), the goal should be: "Mr. Jones will increase his bilateral upper extremity (BUE) strength from poor to normal."

"Measurable" indicates that the goal should be measured in some way. This could be added to Mr. Jones's goal by stating that his muscle strength will be tested by the manual muscle test (MMT). Some therapists may also use a dynamometer to provide an objective reading of muscle strength.

A goal must be "attainable"; if it isn't, it will only frustrate the client and the therapist. In the above example, increasing Mr. Jones's arm strength from poor to normal is not realistically attainable within a short

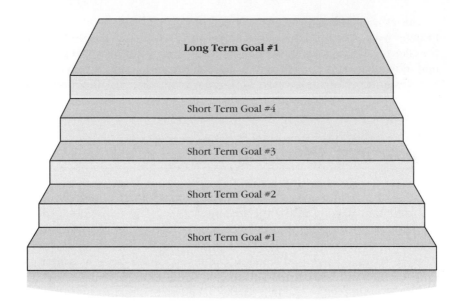

Figure 7-9. Specific short-term goals (STG) are the steps leading up to the broader long-term goals (LTG).

period of time. A more attainable, and therefore more appropriate, goal would be: "Mr. Jones will increase his BUE strength from poor to fair minus" (see Figure 7–5).

A "realistic" goal is also very important. If Mr. Jones has had a complete transaction of his cervical spinal cord (i.e., the spinal cord in his neck has been completely severed), it is doubtful that he will regain any muscle strength in his arms.

The last part of the goal is its "timely" application, meaning that each goal must have a time limit imposed for completion. If a time limit or target completion date is not set, the goal may never be achieved. A goal without a time limit is like a teenager responding "later" to a parent asking "When will you be home?"—the answer really doesn't tell us anything.

If we use the S.M.A.R.T. approach to revisit our goal, it should now look something like this: Mr. Jones will increase his BUE overall strength from poor to fair minus (specific), as measured by a dynamometer (measurable), using graduated resistance (attainable and realistic) within four weeks (timely).

The therapist must always keep the client's wishes and desires at the forefront when developing the treatment plan. If the client has no desire to pursue a particular activity or goal, he is not going to be very cooperative; thus, achieving that goal will be difficult, if not impossible.

For example, Mr. Davis lives alone in an apartment. He has never cooked in his life, because his late wife always did the cooking. Because he will be returning home following his discharge from the rehabilitation center, the occupational therapist thinks that it would be good for him to know how to cook. She builds her entire treatment plan around this and related activities. The therapist becomes discouraged and annoyed with Mr. Davis during therapy sessions because he does not actively participate in the activity. She has disregarded his statements that he intends to order food by phone or have friends and family prepare meals for him. The therapist documents that Mr. Davis is "noncompliant" with therapy and discharges him soon after.

It wasn't that Mr. Davis was noncompliant, however—he just wasn't interested in that particular activity. Had the therapist taken the time to find out what his interests were in the first place, the therapy process may have been much smoother. Although the goals devised by the therapist may have been specific, measurable, and timely, they were not realistic; therefore, they were not attainable.

Treatment Frequency

Part of the treatment plan involves determining how often the client will be seen for therapy in order to achieve her goals. The frequency of treatment will vary, depending on where the client is being seen. For example, an inpatient rehabilitation center client may be seen for occupational therapy two or three times each day, five or six days a week, for 45 minutes at a time. In a home health or outpatient setting, the client may only be seen two or three times a week, for one hour at a time.

Treatment frequency is dictated in part by the therapist, in part by the treatment setting, and, in large part, by the third-party payer (such as Medicare or a private insurance company).

The Treatment Process

Once the evaluation has been performed, and the goals and frequency of treatment have been established, the actual treatment sessions can begin. Here, the occupational therapist and occupational therapy assistant have a great deal of latitude in terms of the activities that can be used to meet the goals of therapy.

Let us assume, for example, that one of the goals is to increase the strength and dexterity in the client's hands. The therapist may choose to provide the client with therapy putty (similar to Silly Putty®) and instruct him in specific exercises to both strengthen hand muscles and increase finger dexterity.

The same therapist may decide that the therapy putty might be boring for another client working toward the same goal, and may instead engage her in a knitting activity, which will also strengthen her hand muscles and increase fine motor skills. This activity may be more appealing to this particular client, because she has always enjoyed knitting in the past.

Still another client may achieve the same goal by participating in a ceramic activity. The pliability and resistance of the clay is similar to that of therapy putty, but the client will have a finished product at the end of the session rather than simply putting the therapy putty back into its container.

If properly planned and executed, the occupational therapy process can engage the client in activities that are fun, meaningful, educational, and therapeutic. The problem with this utopian ideal is that many people will later complain that "we really didn't do any therapy, we just played games and did crafts." This is the blessing and the curse of the profession. It is sometimes necessary to explain to the client how the therapeutic process has helped her to increase her strength, range of motion, endurance, and fine motor skills, which now allow her to participate in activities of daily living and to live a more independent life.

Children, of course, expect to play. Occupational therapy treatment sessions with children frequently resemble nothing more than play sessions. However, in the course of these "play sessions," the child may be learning and incorporating many necessary skills to help him function both in school and at home. Things that most of us take for granted can be addressed, such as sitting and standing, balance, the ability to attend to stimuli, the ability to reach across one's body and grab something on the opposite side (crossing midline), or even something as simple as holding one's head up in order to eat a snack.

All activities chosen by the therapist must ultimately have therapeutic implications. It is not therapeutic to perform passive range of motion exercises on someone with full active range of motion and normal strength. All activities must be performed in order to achieve a specific goal or goals. All activities must be appropriate for the individual based on such factors as age, educational level, cultural values, and personal interests.

Activities must also be graded, from easy to difficult, based on the client's current (and ever-changing) level of ability. This is very important to the success of the therapy program; if an activity is too easy, the client will become bored, and if an activity is too difficult, the client will become frustrated. In either case, the client will not want to participate in that activity. Both the therapist and the client must be aware of goals that are too ambitious, as they can result in frustration and failure.

Throughout the treatment process, the occupational therapist or occupational therapy assistant must constantly monitor the goals. The therapist will frequently modify a goal, change it, or eliminate it altogether. As goals are achieved, new ones may be added to replace them, or therapy can continue to focus on the remaining goals. When all of the goals have been achieved, the client is ready to be discharged.

Discharging the Client from Therapy

When all of the occupational therapy goals have been met, or if the client cannot or will not participate in therapy, the client is ready to be discharged. A client may be discharged from one level of care, such as an acute care hospital, to another level of care, such as home health, an inpatient rehabilitation center, an outpatient rehabilitation center, or a long-term care facility. It is possible, and likely, that the client will resume occupational therapy services at that new level of care.

The client may no longer be appropriate for any type of therapy, due to rapidly declining physical or mental functioning. In cases such as this, the occupational therapist can educate the client's caregivers on ways to better care for the client. It is also not unusual, particularly in the case of hospice, for the patient to die.

SUMMARY

This chapter has presented a generic overview of the occupational therapy process (Figure 7-10 provides a schematic view of this process). Each occupational therapy treatment plan is individualized for the specific client being treated.

The chapter began by presenting how occupational therapy services are requested via a physician's order or through the school system. The evaluation process was described, including the use of the occupational history, temporal adaptation assessment, interest inventory, and caregiver assessment.

The physical assessment was next addressed; this includes the evaluation of areas including muscle strength, joint mobility, active and passive range of motion, gross and fine motor functioning, and sensory testing.

Cognitive and perceptual assessments were also addressed. These assessments include testing an individual's intellectual functioning and how she thinks, learns, understands, and judges. Perception is the

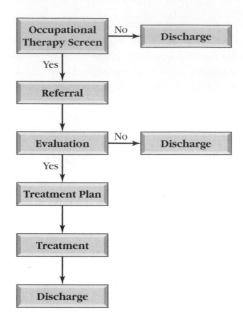

Figure 7-10. Occupational therapy treatment process schematic diagram.

recognition and interpretation of sensory stimuli that serve as a basis for understanding, learning, and knowing.

Activities of daily living are the next assessment area, which include dressing, bathing, eating, food preparation, home management, and work skills, among others.

The treatment planning process includes the development of short- and long-term goals that are specific, measurable, attainable, realistic, and timely (S.M.A.R.T.). A short-term goal is limited in its duration and, combined with other short-term goals, eventually leads to the achievement of the broader long-term goal(s).

The treatment used in occupational therapy must be of interest to the client, and the treatment process itself must be flexible enough to change as the client's needs and desires dictate. Finally, the client must be discharged from therapy when the goals have been achieved, or when the client cannot or will not participate in the therapeutic process any longer.

References

Brinkman, R., & Kirschner, R. (1990). *Dealing with difficult people.* Denver, CO: Career Track Audio.

Geschwind, N. (1975). The apraxias: Neural mechanisms of disorders of learned movement. *Scientific American, 63,* 168.

Marcil, W. M., & Tigges, K. N. (1992). *The person with AIDS: A personal and professional perspective.* Thorofare, NJ: Slack, Inc.

Matsutsuyu, J. S. (1969). The interest check list. *American Journal of Occupational Therapy, 23*(4), 323–328.

Moorhead, L. (1969). The occupational history. *American Journal of Occupational Therapy, 23*(4), 329–334.

Mosby's medical, nursing, and allied health dictionary (5th ed.) (1998). St. Louis, MO: Mosby.

Tigges, K. N., & Marcil, W. M. (1988). *Terminal and life-threatening illness: An occupational behavior perspective.* Thorofare, NJ: Slack, Inc.

Trombly, C. A., & Podolski, C. R. (2002). Assessing abilities and capacities: Range of motion, strength, and endurance. In C. A. Trombly & M. V. Radomski (Eds.), *Occupational therapy for physical dysfunction* (5th ed., p. 83). Philadelphia, PA: Lippincott Williams & Wilkins.

Wheatley, C. J. (2001). Evaluation and treatment of cognitive dysfunction. In L. W. Pedretti & M. B. Early (Eds.), *Occupational therapy practice skills for physical dysfunction* (pp. 444–445). St. Louis, MO: Mosby.

CHAPTER 8

Diseases and Disorders Occupational Therapists Frequently Treat

Chapter Goals

At the conclusion of this chapter, the reader should:

- Be familiar with the developmental disorders occupational therapists treat.
- Be familiar with the mental disorders occupational therapists treat.
- Be familiar with the physical disorders occupational therapists treat.
- Have a basic understanding of the occupational therapy process for each disorder.
- Understand the concept of disease comorbidity.

INTRODUCTION

This chapter will describe the various diseases and disorders that are frequently seen and treated by occupational therapists and occupational therapy assistants.

*This is by no means an exhaustive list, and it should be noted that oc-
cupational therapy services can be utilized by people with virtually any
disability or disorder.*

*To make your life a little bit easier, I have divided these disorders into
three main sections: developmental disorders, mental disorders, and
physical disorders. Each section will present the material in alphabetical
order and give an overview of each condition. I will then present an
overview of possible occupational therapy intervention for each disorder; however, although the signs and symptoms of any given disease or
disability may be similar, each person is different and intervention
must be custom designed for the individual client. Similarly, every
therapist is different, and although the overall intervention process is a
constant, individual therapists will likely put their own spin on the pro-
ceedings. There is no cookbook for occupational therapy intervention—
there are only guidelines.*

*This chapter does not go into great detail, and I would encourage you
to consult more advanced texts or specific Web sites for more detailed information. Having said that, however, some of the terminology in this
chapter is kind of challenging, but it is difficult to avoid its use.*

*The conditions and disorders covered in this chapter do not neces-
sarily occur independently of other conditions, and many individuals
frequently suffer from multiple problems (Figure 8–1). For example, a
man currently being treated for a stroke may also have a number of
other physical problems at the same time; this is known as comorbidity.
This man may be overweight and have diabetes, both of which may
have contributed to his stroke. This same man may also present with*

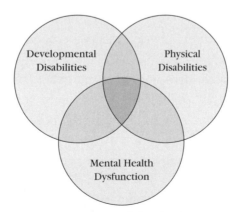

Figure 8-1. The interaction between physical, developmental, and
mental disabilities. Life is often complicated.

*symptoms of clinical depression, which may or may not have been pres-
ent before his stroke. To add further insult to injury, the individual may
have the added burden of mental retardation. The intersection of physical, mental, and developmental disabilities can, and does, occur on a
regular basis.*

*Most occupational therapists and occupational therapy assistants
tend to specialize in one particular area. Therefore, the following list is
not meant to imply that any given therapist would be prepared to work
with all of these disorders.*

Developmental Disorders

Developmental disorders are those conditions with which children are
either born, known as congenital disabilities or birth defects, or that they
acquire during childhood and early adolescence. In the past, many of
these children would have died; those who managed to survive would
often be placed in institutions to live out their lives in a meaningless, day-
to-day existence. With advancements in modern medical care, the survival
rates of developmentally impaired children have increased dramatically.
Furthermore, interventions by allied health personnel, including occupational therapists, have helped to increase the quality of life not only for
these children, but for their families as well.

The types of developmental disabilities and disorders are vast and varied. Each child must be evaluated as an individual, and her needs should
be determined by the occupational therapist (who makes up one part of
the health care or rehabilitation team). The child and her family should
also be made an integral part of that team.

Attention-Deficit Hyperactivity Disorder

Attention-deficit hyperactivity disorder (ADHD) is a behavioral disorder
characterized by inattention, hyperactivity, and impulsivity severe enough
to impair the child's ability to attend to a given activity. These children
are typically considered challenging to supervise, and they frequently run
into problems in social situations, particularly in the school setting. On
the positive side, children with ADHD are often extremely creative,
because they able to "think outside the box."

This diagnosis is, however, somewhat controversial; many people think
that ADHD is over-diagnosed and that too many children are medicated in
an attempt to keep them under control, while simultaneously stifling their
creativity. Thus, the jury is still out on this diagnosis and treatment.

Occupational therapy intervention for a child with ADHD may include sensorimotor training by means of sensory integrative techniques to help the child calm down and better attend to instructions and details. Other possible areas that the occupational therapist might address include fine motor training, eye-hand coordination training, reducing impulsive behaviors, and following instructions (Reed, 2001).

Autism Spectrum Disorders

Autism spectrum disorders (ASD), also known as pervasive developmental disorders (PDD), are a group of disorders affecting children that are characterized by impaired communication and social skills, accompanied by stereotyped behaviors such as rocking, head-banging, and self-injurious behaviors (National Institute of Mental Health, 2004).

The most severe form of this disorder, autism disorder, is marked by poor social and interaction skills, impaired receptive and expressive communication skills, and repetitive behaviors in the form of obsessive preoccupation with certain activities and difficulty with changes in routine.

A milder form of autism is Asperger's syndrome (AS). Children with AS tend to have normal to above-normal intelligence, but they have difficulty with social skills and exhibit obsessive interest in specific areas and certain routines. They tend to have difficulty reading others' moods and body language as well, often leading to awkward social interactions.

Occupational therapy intervention for ASD may also include a sensory integrative approach to help stimulate the child or calm him down, depending on his needs. Specific areas of attention may include developing play skills, interaction skills, communication skills, and general activity of daily living (ADL) independence (Reed, 2001). The therapist should be careful not to overload the child, because this will cause him to become agitated and shut down.

Rett syndrome (RS), a rare autism spectrum disorder, is a genetic developmental disorder that disproportionately affects girls. The newborn appears to be normal in appearance and development. Between the ages of 6–18 months, however, noticeable changes occur, including the slowing of head circumference growth, impaired expressive language, loss of purposeful hand movements, repetitive non-purposeful hand movements, and impaired ability to walk. Other symptoms include low muscle tone (**hypotonia**), disinterest in play activity, autistic-like symptoms, mental retardation, muscle wasting, and **scoliosis** (a lateral, or sideways, curvature of the spine).

Occupational therapy intervention can be extremely important to a child with RS. The focus of treatment (in conjunction with speech pathology) can include hand-to-mouth activities to simulate feeding and swallowing (Reed, 2001). Any sensory stimulating activity is important, and getting the child to pick up and manipulate objects in a meaningful way should be part of the treatment process. Other areas of focus might include training in bathing and dressing skills.

Cancer/Leukemia

Perhaps no other childhood disease is more feared than a diagnosis of cancer. Each year, almost 17,000 children are diagnosed with some type of cancer; of these, 35%—or 5,000—will die, despite the vast improvements in modern treatment. The current treatments for cancer include surgery, chemotherapy, and radiation therapy, all of which can severely impact the child and her family.

We have all seen pictures of children undergoing treatment for cancer, particularly leukemia. We may see them with bald heads, going to Disney World or other places courtesy of the Make-A-Wish Foundation, and our hearts go out to them. Trips like these are undertaken in order to make life worthwhile to the terminally or seriously ill child. We want these children to enjoy life as much as possible, rather than live every day with the specter of pain, discomfort, and death over their heads.

Occupational therapy can also help in this regard. By engaging these children in their primary occupational performance area of play (and as students), the occupational therapist or occupational therapy assistant can help to keep the child strong, vital, and independent to some degree. Those of you who have seen the movie *Patch Adams* (which I recommend very highly) may remember the scene where Patch goes into the children's ward, dresses up as a clown, and makes the children laugh. In the movie, this made a big difference in those children's lives. In real life, too, play, laughter, and a feeling of personal investment in any activity can have a positive impact on one's immune system and, in many cases, can literally mean the difference between life and death.

Cerebral Palsy

Cerebral palsy (CP) is the most common cause of disability in children. It results from damage to the brain either before birth (prenatal), during the birthing process (perinatal), and after birth (postnatal). Any child who sustains a serious head injury with subsequent physical impairments, between birth and 12 years of age, is considered to have cerebral palsy.

Brain damage can be caused by a variety of conditions, such as anoxia (loss of oxygen to the brain), bleeding in the brain, maternal infection during pregnancy, difficult or prolonged labor, forceps delivery, brain tumor, or head trauma. The specific part of the brain that is damaged will determine the types of symptoms that will be present; speech and cognitive functioning may or may not be involved.

There are three main types of cerebral palsy: spastic, athetoid, and ataxic. **Spastic** cerebral palsy tends to result in excessive muscle tone, which can cause either excessive flexion or extension of the arms and legs. Without therapeutic intervention, children with this type of cerebral palsy can develop **contractures** (shortening of muscles) of their joints, resulting in limitations in movement.

With **athetoid** cerebral palsy, the child exhibits almost constant involuntary movements in the form of facial grimacing and slow, writhing movements of the arms (and sometimes the legs). Stress and emotion can increase these involuntary muscle movements.

The child with **ataxic** cerebral palsy typically has poor balance and uncoordinated movement of the arms and legs, which makes walking and self-care difficult. The severity of each type of cerebral palsy will vary from person to person, but all will have some degree of disability.

Occupational therapy intervention will depend on the type and severity of the cerebral palsy, as well as the needs and wants of the individual client. Many children (and adults) require special positioning in wheelchairs to allow them to participate in daily activities, such as eating or taking notes in class. Others may require splints on their hands to prevent contractures or promote function. Still others may require special neurophysiologic exercise regimens to help normalize muscle tone.

Occupational therapists also specialize in adapting toys for children with cerebral palsy (and other developmental disorders), so that the children can control them independently. This adaptation frequently involves remote control devices, large switches, or even toys that can be controlled by eye movements.

Developmental Delay

Developmental delay is a term used to describe the failure of a child to reach **developmental milestones,** such as height and weight appropriate for her age group. Developmental milestones are a series of age-specific criteria that compare a given child to thousands of her peers. For example, by six months of age, a child should be able to sit up with a little bit of support. By 12 months of age, a child should be able to pull herself up and stand briefly without support. By 18 months of age, a child should be able to walk without help (oddly enough, all three of my children could run and climb at the same time, and I longed for the days of sitting with a bit of support). These milestones are merely averages or norms (Figure 8–2); a child who is late in achieving, or fails to achieve, these milestones is considered developmentally delayed.

AGE	MILESTONE
1 month	Picks head up in prone position Visually follows stimuli
2 months	Smiles Recognizes mother
6 months	Sits unsupported
10 months	Pulls up to standing position
12 months	Walks unaided Uses cup and spoon
18 months	Walks up stairs
24 months	Walks down stairs
3 years	Dresses
5 years	Ties

Figure 8-2. Some examples of normal developmental disabilities.

The child who is disabled may reach these milestones late, or not at all. Occupational therapy can help, however, by gearing activities to allow the child to reach some of them. We have little control over a child's height and weight, but milestones such as turning over and sitting up can be worked toward.

Down Syndrome

Down syndrome, also known as trisomy 21 and mongolism, is a disorder caused by a defect of chromosome 21. People with Down syndrome have a distinctive appearance, including slanting, almond-shaped eyes (giving rise to the now politically incorrect term "mongoloid"), a small mouth, and a protruding tongue. Additionally, these individuals typically have intelligence quotients (IQs) between 30 and 50 (Professional Guide to Diseases, 2005).

Although these children have intelligence in the mild to severe range of mental retardation, many of them are educable. Occupational therapy can focus on daily living skills such as bathing, dressing, and house-keeping. Vocational skills can also be addressed, allowing many of these individuals to find work in vocational programs or other areas.

Occupational therapy for the client with Down syndrome varies in approach. Self-care activities, such as bathing and dressing, are important to help the individual become more independent in performing ADLs.

Feeding activities may be addressed as well, because many people with Down syndrome have an uncontrolled tongue thrust that may interfere with eating.

Depending on the level of mental retardation present, it may be difficult to teach the individual ADL skills. Sometimes it may be necessary to employ the teaching techniques of **forward chaining** or **backward chaining.** Forward chaining involves teaching a task in order, from the beginning to the end. This is the way that most people learn how to perform almost any task that is new to them. Backward chaining, as you may have guessed, is the process of teaching a task from its finished state or final steps, backward.

For example, if one was to learn how to put on a shirt using the forward chaining technique, one would pick the shirt up, place it in the proper orientation (with the tag in the back), slide one's arms into the appropriate sleeves, put one's head through the neck hole, and pull it over the head.

Teaching this same task using the backward chaining technique would involve starting with the shirt completely on the torso, pulling one's head out of the neck hole, removing one arm and then the next from the sleeves, pulling the shirt completely off, and laying the shirt down on the bed. The backward chaining technique is usually used with people who have a very low level of intelligence.

Epidermolysis Bullosa

Epidermolysis bullosa (EB) is a rare, hereditary group of blistering skin conditions that causes the skin to blister easily and, in many cases, to slough off, leaving open areas on the skin that are extremely painful and prone to infection. As the skin continually regenerates, it can sometimes cause the fingers and toes to become fused together, making object manipulation and fine motor tasks difficult or impossible. Limitations of other joints, such as the elbows and shoulders, are also possible due to the constant sloughing and regeneration of the skin.

Individuals with EB must frequently have the open lesions (sores) covered in medicated gauze that needs to be changed every few days. This process can be time consuming and painful.

The occupational therapist can assist these individuals by educating them in the use of assistive devices to make daily activities easier and by adapting the individual's environment to promote function and independence. Items like the **universal cuff,** which aids them in holding objects such as eating utensils, toothbrushes, and other self-care devices, can be very helpful to these individuals. Adapting pens or computer keyboards to help the individual write and type more easily can also be helpful.

Failure to Thrive

Failure to thrive (FTT) is a condition in which a child, age two or younger, does not gain weight or grow and remains below height and weight in her age group. The causes of FTT can be organic in nature, such as congenital disorders or diseases including cystic fibrosis, diabetes, and HIV infection. Nonorganic causes include poor nutrition, child abuse, and neglect (Denton, 1986).

"Failure to thrive" typically refers to the child's retarded growth and usually does not address abnormal emotional, intellectual, or social development, although these may occur with FTT.

Occupational therapy intervention for FTT typically focuses on the child's play and feeding skills, along with interpersonal interactions. Denton (1986) has recommended evaluating the child's overall responsiveness, level of irritability, posturing and movement patterns, and deficiencies in oral-motor functions. Development of gross and fine motor skills can lead to increased strength, endurance, and participation in activities.

Fetal Alcohol Spectrum Disorder

Fetal Alcohol Spectrum Disorders include Fetal Alcohol Syndrome (FAS), Fetal Alcohol Effects (FAE), Partial Fetal Alcohol Effects (pFAE), Alcohol Related Neurodevelopmental Disorders (ARND), Static Encephalopathy (SE), and Alcohol-Related Birth Defects (ARBD). All of these disorders are caused by a woman's consumption of alcohol while she is pregnant. The extent of the damage is related to the amount of alcohol consumed during pregnancy. Alcohol consumption during pregnancy is the leading cause of birth defects in the United States—it is also the most preventable.

The most serious of these conditions is Fetal Alcohol Syndrome. The child with FAS may exhibit low birth weight, failure to thrive, developmental delay, facial abnormalities, seizures, poor coordination and fine motor skills, learning disabilities, poor reasoning and judgment skills, and social and behavioral problems. Later in life, these children are at risk for psychiatric problems, criminal behavior, and unemployment.

The most important role for the occupational therapist is prevention, by educating pregnant women and potentially pregnant women about the dangers of alcohol consumption during pregnancy; prevention is paramount.

Fragile X Syndrome

Fragile X syndrome is a hereditary/genetic disorder that results from damage to the X chromosome. You may recall that males have an X and a Y chromosome, and females have two X chromosomes; therefore, the symptoms of Fragile X syndrome will be different among males and females.

The symptoms of Fragile X syndrome include mental retardation, autism, hyperactivity, and a neurological condition known as Fragile X-associated tremor ataxia syndrome (FXTAS) that affects balance, coordination, and memory.

For the occupational therapist working with a child with Fragile X syndrome, the treatment approach would be similar to that taken with a child with autism or mental retardation. Sensory-integrative techniques would be utilized to normalize muscle tone and attention, and activities may revolve heavily around play. If the child has FXTAS, the therapist might utilize weighted toys and utensils to decrease the tremors that may occur during activities.

HIV/AIDS

The human immunodeficiency virus (HIV), the virus that causes AIDS, was unheard of until the early 1980s; by the end of that decade, the first HIV-positive babies were being born, primarily to drug-addicted mothers, prostitutes, or both. HIV is a virus that destroys the body's ability to fight off infection. This inability to protect the body eventually leads to severe illness and death if no treatment is provided.

A woman can transmit HIV to her child during pregnancy, during labor and delivery, and even after the baby is born (through breast milk). Although most babies born to HIV-infected mothers may initially test HIV positive, after about 15 to 18 months many will seroconvert, or test negative.

Children who are HIV positive are likely to be frequently ill with both normal childhood infections, such as inner ear infections and colds, and opportunistic infections—that is, infections that typically do not affect someone with a normally functioning immune system.

Due to the strain on the child's body from this lack of immune protection, he may experience failure to thrive, developmental delay, seizures, cerebral palsy, and mental retardation. In short, due to an improperly functioning immune system, almost anything that can go wrong is possible.

Mental Retardation

Mental retardation (MR) is a syndrome of subnormal intellectual development that can impact learning and social behaviors (Professional Guide to Diseases, 2005). Mental retardation has many causes and may

IQ	DESCRIPTION
10–24	Profound Mental Retardation
25–39	Severe Mental Retardation
40–54	Moderate Mental Retardation
55–69	Mild Mental Retardation
70–84	Borderline
85–99	Low Average
100–114	Average
115–124	High Average
125–129	Superior
130–140	Very Superior/Gifted

Figure 8-3. Ranges of IQ

frequently accompany other conditions, such as cerebral palsy, Down syndrome, and pregnancy complications.

Mental retardation is determined by intelligence tests, such as the Stanford-Binet Intelligence Scale, and its severity is determined by the individual's IQ. Figure 8–3 outlines the various levels of intelligence by score and diagnostic level.

Occupational therapy intervention for a client with mental retardation may focus on self-care activities such as bathing, dressing, simple meal preparation, and basic household tasks. If the client is involved in a vocational program, the occupational therapist may focus on work-related activities by making the work environment user-friendly and providing appropriate equipment to help facilitate the work. Much of the teaching process may involve the forward chaining/backward-chaining approach discussed earlier.

Muscular Dystrophy

The muscular dystrophies are a group of genetic diseases characterized by progressive weakness and degeneration of skeletal muscles (National Institute of Neurological Disorders and Stroke, 2005). Muscular dystrophy (MD) causes weakness in the muscles and wasting, or atrophy, of the muscle tissue, making movement difficult or impossible. Although there are a number of different types of MD, this section will focus on the most common childhood types: myotonic muscular dystrophy, Duchenne muscular dystrophy, Becker muscular dystrophy, and limb-girdle muscular dystrophy.

Myotonic muscular dystrophy is characterized by muscle spasms in the fingers, face, and feet, which cause the individual to walk with a high-stepping gait that is necessary to allow the feet to clear the ground. Myotonic MD can occur at any point in one's life, from early childhood to adulthood, and is considered to be the most common form of adult MD (Muscular Dystrophy Association, 2005). In addition to the muscle weakness, there can also be heart problems and a condition of the eyes known as cataracts, which causes the lenses of the eyes to cloud up and impair vision.

Facioscapulohumeral muscular dystrophy typically affects children between 10 and 15 years old. The disease primarily causes weakness in the face, shoulders, and arms (hence, the name), but it can affect leg muscles as well.

Perhaps the most common form of MD is Duchenne muscular dystrophy, which typically affects boys between the ages of two and six. When most people think of MD, this is what they think of; the muscles of the pelvis and legs are initially affected, causing the child to walk with a waddling gait and frequently on the tips of his toes. Eventually, other muscles are affected, and most children with Duchenne have to rely on wheelchairs for mobility. As the child gets older, he may develop heart and breathing problems. Most children who survive to adulthood will die by the age of 30.

Becker MD is very similar to Duchenne MD, although the age of onset is later, and the person is usually able to walk until his 30s.

Finally, limb-girdle muscular dystrophy (LGMD) can affect boys and girls, and usually strikes in adolescence or early adulthood. This form of MD begins in the hips and moves to the shoulders, causing weakness of the arms and legs. Within 20 years of onset, the individual will have extreme difficulty walking and will probably require a wheelchair.

Prenatal Exposure to Toxins

A pregnant woman must be extremely careful about what she eats, drinks, swallows, and breathes, for the sake of her unborn baby. Everything that the mother ingests can have a serious impact on the development of the fetus. Any substance that interferes with normal prenatal development is called a **teratogen.** Examples of teratogens include drugs and chemicals (particularly alcohol), maternal infections such as rubella and cytomegalovirus, and maternal conditions including diabetes mellitus and lupus (Mosby's Medical, Nursing, and Allied Health Dictionary, 1998).

The effects of a teratogen can result in conditions such as fetal alcohol syndrome, mental retardation, cerebral palsy, or malformation of limbs and organs. In short, any substance that interferes with any stage in the development of a child will result in some type of birth defect.

Occupational therapy interventions with children who suffer from the effects of teratogens will vary from child to child, and will depend upon the specific problems that the child might have. These defects may be obvious and visible, such as a missing limb, or they may be more subtle, such as mental retardation.

A famous example of a teratogen occurred in the 1960s, when many pregnant women around the world took the sedative thalidomide. The birth defects caused by thalidomide were numerous, depending upon the fetus's stage of development when the mother took the drug. The most common birth defect associated with thalidomide was the stunted growth of arms and legs, along with missing or webbed fingers and toes. Occupational therapists had to help these children learn how to function with what limbs they had or, in some cases, teach them how to use prosthetic limbs instead.

Shaken Baby Syndrome

Shaken baby syndrome (SBS) is a tragic sign of our times. Perhaps the most heinous type of child abuse, SBS occurs when an infant, typically 12 months old or younger, is violently shaken back and forth by an adult (usually for crying), causing whiplash-like injuries to the child's head and neck that may include bleeding within the skull, swelling of the brain, and bleeding in the retina of the eye (Poskey, 2005).

The damage resulting from this is serious. If the child survives (approximately 30% of victims die), he will most likely be partially or completely blind, be dependent on others for most areas of self-care, and have cerebral palsy, failure to thrive, and developmental delay. The extent of the injuries will determine the approach that needs to be taken by the occupational therapist or occupational therapy assistant.

Sickle Cell Disease

Sickle cell disease, sometimes called sickle cell anemia, is a hereditary disease that causes normally rounded red blood cells to become deformed and replaced by hard, sticky, sickle-shaped cells that block the normal flow of blood, resulting in pain, damage, and anemia (The Sickle Cell Information Center, 2005). Sickle cell disease is most prominent among African Americans but can also occur in people of Mediterranean descent, including Arabs, Greeks, Italians, and Indians. The sickle cell trait is a defense against malaria; if one parent carries the trait and the other does not, the child is protected against malaria. However, when both parents carry the trait, the offspring develops sickle cell disease, which is not beneficial.

Complications of sickle cell disease include pain (especially in joints), strokes, increased infections, jaundice, kidney damage, anemia, and delayed growth.

Spina Bifida

Spina bifida is a disorder caused by the incomplete closure of one or more of the lower back (lumbosacral) vertebrae during the first three months of pregnancy. The severity of this problem can range from minimal with few symptoms (spina bifida occulta) to severe (myelomeningocele), resulting in paralysis and bowel and bladder problems.

Occupational therapy intervention for a child with spina bifida may include upper-extremity strengthening to compensate for lower-extremity weakness or paralysis, bowel and bladder training, and adaptive equipment acquisition and education. The focus of treatment is on increasing the child's independence in occupational performance areas, particularly self-care and work (school) skills.

Sensory Integrative Disorder

Sensory integration disorder (SID) is a blanket term used to describe conditions that cause a child (or adult) to have difficulty integrating, or making sense of, the stimuli entering the brain from the five senses of vision, smell, taste, hearing, and touch. Sensory integrative disorders may be seen in conditions such as autism spectrum disorders, cerebral palsy, attention-deficit hyperactivity disorder, and anxiety disorders.

The child with SID may exhibit a variety of symptoms, including sensitivity to sound, light, certain food textures, or touch (tactile defensiveness); delayed speech and motor skills; and problems with motivation and social interactions, among many others.

Sensory integration disorder is a condition that was recognized and named by an occupational therapist, the late A. Jean Ayres, in the 1970s. From her research, Ayres developed a therapeutic frame of reference based upon sensory integration—to help effectively integrate renegade sensations in order to facilitate normal function in the child and, consequently, allow him to participate in activities such as schoolwork, self-care skills, and play activities.

Sensory integration activities include those that stimulate or inhibit the central nervous system (CNS) by means of the five senses, as well as by facilitation or inhibition of the **vestibular system,** which is responsible for balance, orientation in space, and posture.

A good example of a sensory integration activity is the use of a hanging net to either stimulate or inhibit a child's vestibular system. If a child is hyperactive and needs to calm down prior to performing an activity, the therapist might place that child in the net and very slowly and gently rock him. If you were trying to calm a baby down and get her to go to sleep, you would gently rock her while she was wrapped in a warm blanket; you might even sing softly to her in a darkened or dimly lit room. These are all inhibitory techniques used by sensory integration therapists.

On the other hand, if the child requires facilitation in order to become more alert or increase muscle tone, the therapist might rock him quickly and spin him in the net; this is a facilitory technique. If you think about what it is like to ride on a roller coaster, you know that it is impossible to be very tired or fall asleep on one. When you get off the ride, you are exhilarated. This is another way that vestibular stimulation works.

Children with sensory integrative disorders have difficulty dealing with the sensations that they experience on a daily basis; bright lights, loud noises, or the feeling of a clothing tag against their skin are enough to make these children extremely uncomfortable and upset. The occupational therapist works with the child to help modulate these sensations so that she is able to deal with them appropriately.

Tay-Sachs Disease

Tay-Sachs disease, named after Warren Tay and Bernard Sachs, is a genetic disorder that affects children, primarily those of eastern European Jewish ancestry, causing progressive destruction of the CNS. Children born with Tay-Sachs disease appear quite normal until the age of about six months. At this time, the baby "gradually stops smiling, crawling, or turning over, loses its ability to grasp or reach out, and eventually becomes blind, paralyzed and unaware of its surroundings" (March of Dimes, 2005). The disease is fatal to all affected children by the age of five, and there is no cure for the disorder at this time.

Due to the terminal nature of this disease, all therapeutic intervention is essentially palliative in nature; however, because occupational therapy seeks to help people achieve quality of life, it is most certainly suggested for these children and their families. Occupational therapy intervention might include sensory integration, gross motor training, and ADL training. The occupational therapist might also teach the child's parents how to position the child for feeding and how to reinforce the occupational therapy program.

Mental Disorders

The topic of mental illness is an uncomfortable one for most people. Many people will openly talk about a family member with cancer or another physical problem but will rarely, if ever, discuss a personal mental health issue. Yet, according to the National Institute of Mental Health (NIMH), approximately 22% of Americans suffer from some type of mental disorder!

The stigma, or shame, attached to mental illness is a very real one. In 1999, the surgeon general of the United States reported that the stigma of mental illness "is the most formidable obstacle to future progress in the arena of mental illness and health" (Satcher, 1999). Furthermore, Brown and Bradley (2002) found that "while some 50 million Americans will evidence a mental disorder, only one-fourth of them will seek mental health services" (p. 81), primarily because of the stigma attached to it.

Occupational therapists can, and do, work with people with mental health problems—although not in the numbers that they used to. In fact, only about 5% of occupational therapy practitioners currently work in the mental health field. This sad statistic is the result of both poor funding for mental health services and the "revolving door" services for mental health patients; that is, the same people (the chronically mentally ill) return for treatment repeatedly, although they never seem to get any better and, in many cases, actually get worse. New medications also help to relieve the symptoms of mental illness, and patients are now medicated and quickly discharged more often. There is still, however, a real need for more occupational therapists to return to their roots in the mental health field.

Alzheimer's Disease

Perhaps no other condition worries people more than does Alzheimer's disease (AD). This is a chronic, progressive neurological disease that causes shrinking of brain tissue and results in confusion, memory loss, and loss of physical and cognitive functioning. As the condition worsens, the individual essentially loses all sense of who she is and becomes completely dependent on others for safety and basic needs. Maureen Reagan, daughter of former president Ronald Reagan (who suffered from Alzheimer's disease), has called AD "the long good-bye" because the individual has no sense of identity but continues to exist for many years.

I have included Alzheimer's disease under mental health disorders primarily because of the strong dementia component, with accompanying psychiatric components. However, a significant physical disability component also exists with this condition, including muscle weakness, loss of voluntary muscle control, and increased fatigue.

Anxiety Disorders

Anxiety is a feeling of unease or dread that something bad is about to happen, resulting in apprehension, restlessness, or tension. An individual with anxiety may fidget, pace, and be unable to focus or concentrate.

We all experience anxiety at one time or another; every student has experienced test anxiety at least once, many a prospective bride or groom has experienced "cold feet" prior to the big day, and a number of people would rather have a tooth pulled without anesthesia than speak in front of a crowd (fear of public speaking, by the way, is the number one fear of most people). Anxiety is normal, and, in many cases, it can be beneficial. It becomes a problem, however, when it interferes with an individual's ability to function in her daily life.

Anxiety disorders include panic attacks, agoraphobia (fear of public places), social phobia, specific phobias (such as ornithophobia, the fear of birds), obsessive compulsive disorder (OCD), post-traumatic stress disorder (PTSD), and generalized anxiety disorder (GAD).

Once diagnosed, anxiety disorders can be treated with certain medications, including selective serotonin reuptake inhibitors (SSRIs) such as Luvox®. Medication can help many people break the grip of anxiety and learn how to better deal with their situation.

Occupational therapy can help the anxious client by working to break tasks down into smaller, more manageable segments and teaching her how to better manage time. The occupational therapist or occupational therapy assistant can also teach the client relaxation techniques and lifestyle changes to help reduce anxiety-provoking situations.

As a clinician and teacher, I have observed a great deal of anxiety in others. One of the greatest causes of anxiety is the innate desire many people have to do everything perfectly; in the attempt to be perfect, they are never satisfied with what they have accomplished and are constantly reworking everything (in many instances, this leads to nothing getting accomplished). This condition, known as "perfection paralysis," is counterproductive and causes one's anxiety level to rise drastically. One of the simplest things that an occupational therapist can help the anxious client realize is that nothing in life is perfect, and that he should try to be happy with what he is able to accomplish.

Dementia

Dementia is a chronic, progressive disease of the brain that causes personality changes, impaired mental functioning, impaired judgment, confusion, forgetfulness, and poor impulse control (Mosby's Medical, Nursing, and Allied Health Dictionary, 1998). Some dementias, such as those caused by medications, alcohol, and disease, can be reversed; other dementias, such as those seen in Alzheimer's disease, Parkinson's disease, and arterial disease (**vascular dementia**), cannot. Dementia is sometimes used as a catchall term—thus, people are frequently misdiagnosed with this disease (Figure 8–4).

Occupational therapy intervention for the client with dementia will depend upon the severity of the dementia. The client's safety is paramount,

Older people who act a little bit odd are frequently labeled as having dementia, which is increasingly being described as Alzheimer's disease. Many of these people do not, however, have Alzheimer's disease, nor are they demented; they may instead be suffering from a treatable problem, including the following:

- **Depression.** Depression occurrence is four times higher in the elderly, and the symptoms of depression, such as forgetfulness, confusion, sleep problems, and mood disturbances, can mimic those of dementia. If left untreated, clinical depression can progress to pseudo-dementia and eventually become full-blown dementia. It is possible that someone can have both depression and dementia at the same time.

- **Pernicious Anemia.** Pernicious anemia is a condition in older people that results in a deficiency of vitamin B_{12}. As many as 20% of elderly adults suffer from vitamin B_{12} deficiency; this condition can be easily reversed through administration of vitamin B_{12}.

- **Dehydration.** Despite the availability of bottled water, most of us are dehydrated to some degree. This is particularly true of the elderly, because most elderly have a diminished sense of thirst and, therefore, do not drink enough water or other fluids. Dehydration can cause symptoms almost identical to dementia. These symptoms, however, can be reversed by proper hydration.

- **Urinary Tract Infection.** Urinary tract infection (UTI) can cause mental status changes and confusion in the elderly. Sometimes these changes are the only symptoms of a UTI in an elderly individual. With proper treatment, such as appropriate antibiotic therapy, these symptoms will clear up and the individual will return to normal.

Figure 8-4. When Dementia Isn't Dementia

and it is therefore unreasonable to assume that these individuals will be able to live independently. If the dementia is mild, the occupational therapist can help the client establish a daily routine that can easily be followed. Sometimes, signs and Post-it® Notes can help the client remember to do things such as turning off a light switch or closing a door.

As the severity of the dementia worsens, the client will require greater supervision (for safety reasons) and more assistance with activities of daily living. Activities to prevent loss of mobility may be used, along with activities that stimulate the senses, such as baking or ceramics.

At some point, however, the client will not be able to retain much of what is said to him, and therapy recommendations will have to be directed at family and caregivers. Proper positioning, passive range of motion exercises, and sensory stimulation techniques can all be provided by family members.

Dissociative Disorders

Dissociative disorders involve a disruption of "consciousness, memory, identity, or perception of the environment" (American Psychiatric Association, 1994, p. 477). These disorders can include amnesia, sleepwalking, fugue, and multiple personalities. Dissociative conditions are frequently brought on by severe stress with which a person is unable to cope, causing him to try and separate, or dissociate, himself from the stressor.

Dissociative disorders have long been popular fodder for the entertainment industry. *The Three Faces of Eve* (1957) was a popular movie about a woman who had three distinctive personalities: Eve White, Eve Black, and Jane. The collision of these three personalities caused her to seek psychiatric help, and she was eventually "cured" by an astute and caring psychiatrist.

The occupational therapist working with the dissociative personality is likely to focus on time-management skills and routinization to keep the individual focused and grounded. Relaxation training may be indicated as well, as stress can trigger certain personalities to appear. Problems may arise during treatment, because each distinct personality may have completely different needs and interests than the others.

Eating Disorders

Eating disorders occur when there is a disruption in the eating behaviors of an individual. Most eating disorders occur in young females; however, anyone can be at risk of developing this disorder.

The two eating disorders are anorexia nervosa and bulimia nervosa. Although these two disorders can (and do) occur together, they are, in fact, different from each other.

Anorexia nervosa is a disorder in which the individual is so afraid of gaining weight that she does not eat enough food to allow her to do so. When an anorexic looks at her 85-pound body in the mirror, she sees someone who weighs 160 pounds. This misinterpretation of the way one's body appears is called body dysmorphic disorder. An anorexic can lose so much weight that her body will begin to devour itself in order to meet its nutritional requirements. In time, the severe weight loss can cause an imbalance in the body's electrolytes, which can result in muscular impairment, cognitive difficulties, and heart attacks.

Although the best treatment for anorexia is proper medication and psychotherapy, occupational therapy can also help, especially in the area of the client's self-image. Activities such as shopping for food, preparing it, and eating it can be beneficial to the anorexic, as can choosing stylish clothes, dressing appropriately, and applying tasteful makeup.

Bulimia nervosa involves episodes of binge eating followed by efforts to purge the food by means of self-induced vomiting, overuse of laxatives and diuretics, and excessive exercise. All of these purging methods can have dire consequences on the body: regular vomiting can cause damage to the vocal cords and teeth, regular use of laxatives can result in dependence, and overuse of diuretics can result in an electrolyte imbalance.

The occupational therapy intervention for bulimia is similar to that of anorexia, including shopping for nutritious food, preparing it, and eating it. Activities that help improve body and self-image can also be helpful.

Emotionally Disturbed Children and Adolescents

Serious emotional disturbance, as defined by the Individuals with Disabilities Education Act (IDEA), Public Law 101–476, is

". . . a condition exhibiting one or more of the following characteristics over a long period of time and to a marked degree that adversely affects a child's educational performance.

A. An inability to learn that cannot be explained by intellectual, sensory, or health factors.

B. An inability to build or maintain satisfactory interpersonal relationships with peers and teachers.

C. Inappropriate types of behaviors or feelings under normal circumstances.

D. A general pervasive mood of unhappiness or depression.

E. A tendency to develop physical symptoms or fears associated with personal or school problems." (Federal Register, 1999)

Students with emotional disturbances tend to have difficulty in school for many reasons, including hyperactivity, aggressive behaviors against others or self-injurious behaviors, social withdrawal, immaturity, and learning difficulties.

Occupational therapy intervention for the child with emotional disturbances may include such areas as working in groups, improving gross and fine motor skills, and eye-hand coordination. Following directions and accepting criticism in tasks are also important, as is teaching the child to lose as well as win. In all activities, the child should be encouraged to continue the task regardless of the outcome.

Forensic Psychiatry

"Forensic psychiatry includes a group of disorders that have as their common denominator a person who has entered the criminal justice system because of aggressive, dangerous, or socially unacceptable behavior" (Reed, 2001, p. 798). Forensic psychiatry essentially deals with mentally ill individuals who have been incarcerated for a crime. These individuals may be held in an inpatient facility, such as a maximum security psychiatric hospital, or an outpatient setting. The hospital setting assists the court in determining whether the individual is competent to stand trial and be sentenced for the crime of which he is accused.

The role of the occupational therapist in this setting is typically the same as in any other setting; the difference, however, is that the forensic occupational therapist must be aware of any contraband that the patient may have acquired (such as drugs or weapons), and she contributes to the overall assessment of the individual's level of dangerousness and competency (Victoria Schindler, personal communication, November, 2005). These clients must be assessed and treated on an ongoing basis (Schindler, 2000). Additionally, Stein and Brown (1991) have found that forensic clients benefit most from concrete, reality-based programs.

Mood Disorders

Mood disorders are probably the most common mental illness in the United States today and, possibly, the most unrecognized and untreated. Mood disorders can influence the way a person views herself and the world around her. For our purposes, we will look at the two main mood disorders: clinical depression and bipolar disorder.

Clinical depression is, by far, the most common of all mental illnesses. It is so pervasive that it has been called "the common cold of psychiatry" (Seligman, 1975). Clinical depression affects over 20 million people in the United States at a cost of almost $40 billion per year. Clinical depression also affects women almost three times as often as men.

We all feel sad and out of sorts from time to time: we have a fight with a friend, we lose a beloved pet, friend, or family member, or we feel that others don't understand us. These feelings are normal and, within a short period of time, they pass and we return to our usual selves. For a person suffering from depression, however, these feelings do not go away, and the depressive perceives the world as being against her—nothing ever goes right, and she usually feels that she deserves it. In essence, to the person with depression, every silver lining has a dark cloud.

But depression is more than a mindset; there are physical symptoms, as well. These can include: the inability to sleep (or the opposite, sleeping all of the time); loss of appetite, with corresponding weight loss (or, again, the opposite, excessive eating with excessive weight gain); loss of interest in previously enjoyed activities; boredom; anger with frequent outbursts; constant fatigue; and the inability to concentrate or remember things (Figure 8–5).

The person with depression is unable to motivate himself to do the simplest of tasks. He has difficulty making decisions, and he frequently feels guilty about things that have nothing to do with him. Combined, these factors can seriously impair one's ability to participate effectively in life. Many people with clinical depression are unable to function at their jobs and end up either quitting or being fired. Students with depression cannot focus and often end up failing or dropping out of school.

Appetite disturbance with weight loss or gain

Sleep disturbance

Psychomotor agitation or retardation

Fatigue

Sense of worthlessness

Chronic somatic complaints, such as stomachaches, headaches, dizziness, palpitations, backaches, and paresthesia

Forgetfulness

Inability to concentrate

Figure 8-5. Signs of Depression

Health care professionals need to recognize the symptoms of depression in those for whom they care. Even if we exclude the very real possibility of suicide among many of these individuals, clinical depression can have a serious impact on the client's ability to participate in therapy and can even impair the client's ability to recover from physical disabilities. Numerous screening tools are available to help the clinician recognize depression. Although Figure 8–6 shows only the Geriatric Depression Scale, there are several other depression rating scales available, including the Beck Depression Inventory (BDI), the Zung Self-Rating Depression Scale (SDS), and more.

Bipolar disorder is another mood disorder that can be crippling to those afflicted with it. Previously called **manic depression,** bipolar disorder causes a person to experience extremes in her mood, ranging from

Choose the best answer regarding how you have felt over the past week.

	Yes	No
1. Are you basically satisfied with your life?	Yes	**No**
2. Have you dropped many of your activities or interests?	**Yes**	No
3. Do you feel that your life is empty?	**Yes**	No
4. Do you often get bored?	**Yes**	No
5. Are you in good spirits most of the time?	Yes	**No**
6. Are you afraid that something bad is going to happen to you?	**Yes**	No
7. Do you feel happy most of the time?	Yes	**No**
8. Do you often feel helpless?	**Yes**	No
9. Do you prefer to stay home rather than go out and do new things?	**Yes**	No
10. Do you feel that you have more problems with memory than most?	**Yes**	No
11. Do you think it's wonderful to be alive now?	Yes	**No**
12. Do you feel pretty worthless the way you are now?	**Yes**	No
13. Do you feel full of energy?	Yes	**No**
14. Do you feel that your situation is hopeless?	**Yes**	No
15. Do you think that most people are better off than you?	**Yes**	No

Answers indicating depression are in bold print. Each answer counts as one point; scores greater than five points indicate probable depression.

Source: Sheikh, J. I., & Yesavage, J. A. (1986). Geriatric Depression Scale (GDS): Recent evidence and development of a shorter version. *Clinical Gerontologist, 5,* 165–173. Used by permission.

Figure 8-6. Geriatric Depression Scale (Short Form)

the lowest depths of depression and despair to the highest of highs. These extremes of behavior can be devastating not only to the bipolar person, but also to her family, coworkers, and society at large.

In the manic phase of this illness, the individual may feel that she can do anything at all, with no consequences whatsoever. People in the manic phase frequently go on buying sprees, where they purchase things that they do not need nor can they afford, spending money that they don't have (e.g., making credit card purchases or writing bad checks). They may also engage in substance abuse (using alcohol or street drugs) and promiscuous sexual behavior that can lead to venereal disease or unwanted pregnancy. The individual experiencing extreme mania may hear **auditory hallucinations** (voices in his head) that lead him to do things he normally would not do.

At the other end of the bipolar spectrum—depression—a person may experience exaggerated lows, especially if he has just recently come down from a manic high and now faces the consequences of his actions: credit card bills, the loss of a job, venereal disease, divorce, incarceration, and so forth. Individuals in this state are at high risk for committing suicide, and many do.

Personality Disorders

The personality disorders comprise a relatively large group of relational disorders. Those with personality disorders tend to be rigid and inflexible in their interpersonal relationships, as well as their daily activities. This rigidity makes it difficult for the person to "fit in" among society. As defined by the *Diagnostic and Statistical Manual of Mental Disorders, 4th Edition* (APA, 1994), "A personality disorder is an enduring pattern of inner experience and behavior that deviates markedly from the expectations of the individual's culture, is pervasive and inflexible, has an onset in adolescence or early adulthood, is stable over time, and leads to distress or impairment" (p. 629).

You probably know someone with a personality disorder, although you may not realize it. Many of these individuals may be considered "weird" or some other pejorative. Unfortunately, these people will always be social pariahs, to some extent. Consider the list of personality disorders compiled by the American Psychiatric Association (APA, 1994) and see if you recognize anyone you know.

> **Paranoid personality disorder** is a pattern of distrust and suspiciousness such that other's motives are interpreted as malevolent.
>
> **Schizoid personality disorder** is a pattern of detachment from social relationships and a restricted range of emotional expression.

Schizotypal personality disorder is a pattern of acute discomfort in close relationships, cognitive or perceptual distortions, and eccentricities of behavior.

Antisocial personality disorder is a pattern of disregard for, and violation of, the rights of others.

Borderline personality disorder is a pattern of instability in interpersonal relationships, self-image, affects, and marked impulsivity.

Histrionic personality disorder is a pattern of excessive emotionality and attention seeking.

Narcissistic personality disorder is a pattern of grandiosity, need for admiration, and lack of empathy.

Avoidant personality disorder is a pattern of social inhibition, feelings of inadequacy, and hypersensitivity to negative evaluation.

Dependendent personality disorder is a pattern of submissive and clinging behavior related to an excessive need to be cared for.

Obsessive-compulsive personality disorder is a pattern of preoccupation with orderliness, perfection, and control. (p. 629)

I've known a lot of these people in my lifetime; in fact, I've dated quite a few in the past. Seriously, it should be noted that one person can have multiple personality disorders at the same time, which makes it even more difficult for him to fit into society and establish meaningful relationships.

Occupational therapy intervention with personality disorders will vary according to the individual, the specific personality disorder(s), and the occupational performance area(s) in which the individual is having problems. Bonder (1995), as cited in Reed (2001), stated that the occupational problems caused by personality disorders are derived from four primary issues: "(1) inaccurate perceptions of self and others, (2) inadequate social skills, (3) poorly developed personal values and goals, and (4) poor self-esteem" (p. 812). Occupational therapy intervention, therefore, should address each of these issues as appropriate, in terms of work, self-care, and play and leisure.

Post-Traumatic Stress Disorder

Post-traumatic stress disorder (PTSD) is technically classified as an anxiety disorder (APA, 1994). However, because it is so prevalent in our society, I have given it its own section.

PTSD is a condition that affects an individual who has experienced a terrifying physical or emotional event. This condition was originally seen in soldiers who had experienced combat, and has previously been referred to as shell shock or battle fatigue. The same holds true now, especially in light of our most recent combat veterans. However, many others can experience PTSD as well, following events such as rape, mugging, a motor vehicle accident, or child abuse.

Symptoms of PTSD include sleep disturbances, flashbacks, impaired memory, panic attacks, obsessive behavior, exaggerated startle response, depression, and irritability with occasional violent outbursts. These symptoms can interfere with the individual's ability to interact with others and perform his job effectively.

The ultimate goal of occupational therapy is to get the client to return to as normal a life as possible despite his PTSD. In conjunction with medication and cognitive—or "talk"—therapy, occupational therapy can help these individuals by focusing on "doing" as a way of dealing with the PTSD. Relaxation training and leisure skills training can also help these individuals.

Schizophrenia

When most of us think of mental illness, we think of schizophrenia—and mostly, we think wrong. Schizophrenia is a chronic, progressive brain disorder that affects about 1% of the world's population. In the United States alone, there are approximately 2 million people with schizophrenia. Many of these individuals comprise the hundreds of thousands of homeless people who sleep in subway stations and city parks throughout the country.

Contrary to popular belief, most people with schizophrenia are not violent. Because they have difficulty relating to the "real world," they tend to avoid interacting with others and actually appear to be quite self-absorbed and shy. Another misconception about this disease is that, although the term schizophrenia literally means "split mind," people with schizophrenia do not have "split" or multiple personalities (see dissociative disorders).

One of the goals of occupational therapy is to encourage the client with schizophrenia to appropriately interact with the rest of the world. The client must be able to effectively balance self-care, work, and play and leisure skills so that she can meet her daily goals, beyond merely surviving.

People with schizophrenia often fail to attend to their personal hygiene, which can make them stand out in everyday life. Occupational therapy can help these individuals to realize the importance of daily hygiene and appropriate dress, in order to foster a sense of normalcy in interpersonal interactions.

Occupational therapy is only one part of the total management of schizophrenia, which is a chronic condition. Medication, although not a panacea, is extremely important to these individuals to help them maintain a hold on reality. Many people with schizophrenia stop taking their medication after they are released from the hospital because they "feel better" and do not see the need to continue to take it. Unfortunately, they often end up being rehospitalized because they begin to exhibit bizarre behavior once again.

Self-Injurious Behaviors

Self-injury is the process by which an individual deliberately destroys body tissue by a variety of means, including cutting, carving, scratching, biting, burning or branding, head banging, and hitting. Some argue that excessive tattooing and body piercing (both of which are currently popular) are also forms of self-injurious behavior.

The reasons that people engage in these behaviors can vary from person to person. Many teenagers state that they feel a pressure building up inside of them that can only be relieved through cutting or some similar method. Others state that, by hurting themselves, they are finally able to "feel something." Some do it as a way of gaining attention. Perhaps some are simply masochistic.

Many of these individuals have a problem, be it depression, bipolar disorder, PTSD, or borderline personality disorder. Self-injurious behaviors are also frequently seen in autism spectrum disorder and mental retardation. Those of you who are Harry Potter fans may even recognize that Dobby, the house elf, has a problem with self-injurious behaviors (he repeatedly hits himself and bangs his head against objects when he feels he has misbehaved).

The goal of the occupational therapist working with someone with self-injurious behaviors is to get her to function optimally, in terms of an occupational role, on a daily basis. In the course of therapy, the occupational therapist can suggest alternatives to behaviors such as cutting by substituting less damaging behaviors, such as applying ice to her skin or snapping the skin with a rubber band. These substitutes can help alleviate the need to damage her skin while providing the stimulus that she craves (Anne Burke, personal communication, January, 2006).

Substance Abuse

When we hear the term "substance abuse," many of us tend to think of illegal drugs such as marijuana, cocaine, methamphetamines, and heroin.

However, we can also include other substances such as alcohol (the single most abused substance in the United States and throughout the world), cigarettes, and countless household chemicals that people sniff or huff in an effort to get high.

Why do people want to ingest these things into their bodies? The simple answer to the question is that it makes them feel good, if only for a short while. However, the more frequently the individual uses a given substance, the higher quantity it takes to reach that previous feeling of euphoria, and, subsequently, the individual becomes either physically or psychologically addicted to that substance.

The treatment of substance abuse is a multidisciplinary effort that includes hospitalization, the use of medications, individual and group therapy, and ancillary therapies. Occupational therapy can play an important role by allowing the substance abuser to learn how to better manage his time in a way that does not include alcohol or drugs. Activities that help the client gain mastery over his environment and his use of time can be very empowering to him.

The Role of Occupational Therapy in Mental Health

The role of occupational therapy in mental health disorders is, at once, individualized for each client, while simultaneously aiming for the same goals: 1) to help prepare the client to engage in occupations, 2) to allow the client to effectively plan and use her time, in order to participate in activities of daily living, and 3) to participate in appropriate social interactions. The level of occupational therapy intervention is determined by the level of acuity of the mental illness (Anne Burke, personal communication, January, 2006). For example, the level of intervention for someone who has just had his first psychotic episode will be significantly different than for a person with chronic schizophrenia who routinely skips his medication.

Physical Disabilities

Physical disabilities are the largest group of overall disabilities, and the majority of occupational therapy personnel work with this population. Physical disabilities are acquired and can be brought on by an accident, disease, or age-related changes in the body. Most of us, at some point in our lives, will experience a physical disability, either temporary or permanent.

Amyotrophic Lateral Sclerosis (ALS)

Amyotrophic lateral sclerosis (ALS), also known as Lou Gehrig's disease (after the New York Yankees' first baseman who brought attention to the disease and eventually died from it in 1941), is a neurodegenerative disease that attacks the brain and spinal cord causing muscle weakness, mixed muscle tone (both spasticity and flaccidity), muscle wasting, swallowing problems, and breathing difficulties. As the disease progresses, the individual becomes increasingly weak and incapacitated. Death typically occurs within five years after the onset of symptoms, usually due to the failure of respiratory muscles.

Because ALS is a progressive disease, occupational therapy intervention will depend on the level of disability. Frequently, the client must be positioned so as to maximize function while simultaneously decreasing contractures and pressure sores, or decubidi. People with ALS often have trouble swallowing; therefore, positioning—as well as the consistency and thickness of food—can be very important to prevent choking and the possible development of aspiration pneumonia.

Occupational therapy intervention for clients with ALS is extremely important, and, as the client's condition worsens, it can become vital. The client can be taught an exercise program in the early stages of the disease to prevent loss of strength and range of motion. Splints can be made to help prevent contractures that may occur in the future.

As the client becomes weaker and his muscle strength diminishes, he may require adaptive equipment to help him perform activities such as bathing, dressing, and eating. He may require education in energy conservation and work simplification to help him use his limited energy wisely. Bed and wheelchair positioning become issues, as well, in order to promote function and prevent skin breakdown.

In the final stages of ALS, the client may require more sophisticated devices, such as an environmental control system, to allow him some control over his immediate environment. An environmental control system allows a disabled individual to operate things such as room temperature and lights, and to lock and unlock doors, and so forth, from a remote control unit. Eventually, however, most of these individuals become totally dependent on others for their care.

Amputations

An amputation is the surgical removal of a body part secondary to disease or trauma. The most common cause of amputation is gangrene, which can result from trauma or insufficient blood supply (ischemia).

Other common causes include peripheral vascular disease (PVD), diabetes, frostbite, and burns.

The occupational therapist can teach the client how to wrap his stump and apply his prosthesis. If the client has an upper-extremity amputation, the occupational therapist may help her learn how to apply her prosthesis and how to function while using it. This may include tasks such as self-feeding, dressing, driving a car, or using a pen or keyboard with the prosthesis.

Arthritis

Arthritis, or inflammation of the joints, is probably the most common disabling condition in the world. In fact, most adults over the age of 25 have some degree of arthritis! Arthritis can range in severity from quite mild, causing only occasional pain and discomfort, to so severe that it can incapacitate the individual with pain and deformity, and may even require surgery and joint replacement.

The two main types of arthritis are osteoarthritis and rheumatoid arthritis. **Osteoarthritis** (OA) is, by far, the most common form of arthritis. Also known as **degenerative joint disease** (DJD), osteoarthritis results from wear and tear on the joints and usually takes many years to develop. Commonly affected joints include the fingers, shoulders, hips, and knees. The arthritic hand frequently exhibits deforming bumps of the finger joints, known (depending on their location) as Heberden's nodes or Bouchard's nodes.

Rheumatoid arthritis (RA) is not as common as OA but can be much more devastating. Rheumatoid arthritis is a chronic disease that causes episodes of inflammation and pain in the joints. Over time, the affected joints—particularly the small joints of the fingers and toes—can become severely deformed, making it difficult for the individual to perform the simplest of activities. As the joints of the fingers become unstable, the muscles and tendons of the hand begin to pull bones out of alignment, resulting in deformities of the fingers. Figure 8–7 shows the most common deformities: swan neck deformity, boutonnière deformity, and ulnar drift of the fingers. These deformities can be prevented to some degree by timely intervention, such as the use of splints, and through meticulous attention to joint protection techniques. In severe cases, the affected joints can be replaced by silicone prostheses.

Occupational therapists can be of significant help to people with any type of arthritis. The key to dealing with arthritis is to avoid situations that might aggravate it, which involves a great deal of client education. The client should first be taught **joint protection,** or methods of performing tasks so as not to put any unnecessary strain on the joints, especially

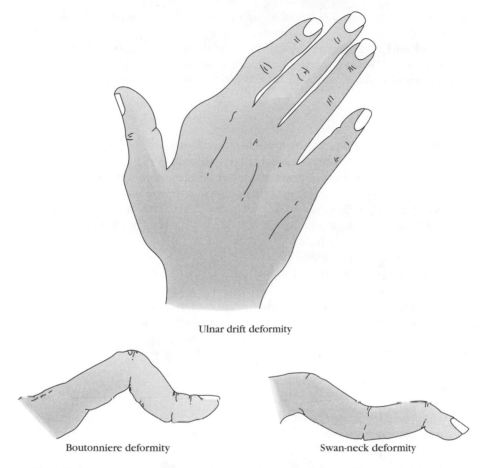

Ulnar drift deformity

Boutonniere deformity   Swan-neck deformity

Figure 8-7. Common joint deformities caused by Rheumatoid arthritis

the smaller joints of the wrist and fingers. Reeducating a client to safely open a jar of peanut butter is an example of joint protection. Normally, when you open a jar, you place all of your fingertips on the edge of the lid and turn. Although this technique is usually effective, it places a great deal of strain on the joints in your wrist and fingers. An alternate method is to place the palm of your hand flat on top of the lid and then turn the lid using your wrist and shoulder. This technique redistributes the force from the smaller joints to larger ones.

The use of **assistive devices** to perform tasks with a minimum of joint strain is another important part of occupational therapy, especially when working with those with arthritis. If we stay with the peanut butter jar example, we can achieve the goal of opening the jar using one of the many types of commercially available jar openers, both manual and electric. Other examples of assistive devices used by people with arthritis include a **sock aid** to allow the individual to put on socks without having to bend over, a **long shoe horn** to put on shoes, and a **dressing stick** to help remove shoes and socks.

Bariatrics

Bariatrics is the branch of medicine that deals with patients who are overweight and the diseases associated with obesity. The U.S. population is growing increasingly larger in physical size; therefore, the field of bariatrics is also growing. People who carry more than 20% of their ideal body weight are considered **obese.** Individuals who are so heavy that they have difficulty breathing are considered **morbidly obese.**

People who are obese often have difficulty performing ADLs and IADLs. Occupational therapists can educate these individuals in the use of assistive devices to help them perform lower extremity dressing, bathing, and personal hygiene, among other things. Foti (2005) stated, "After the problem areas have been identified, the occupational therapist may consider compensatory strategies, adaptive equipment, caregiver training, and resources" (p. 12).

Burns

Serious burns account for more than 300,000 hospitalizations each year; of this number, approximately 6,000 people die as a result of their burns. Many of these victims are children. Burns cause serious physical and psychological scarring and can result in severe loss of function. Burns can be thermal (temperature related), chemical, or electrical in nature, and can be caused by flame, steam, hot liquids, hot metal, radiation (including sunburn), and cold metal.

Burns damage and destroy the skin, the largest single organ in the human body. The skin is the body's first line of defense against infection, and, if seriously damaged, it decreases the body's ability to not only fight infection but to regulate body temperature, as well. The severity of a burn is graded by its depth in the skin (Figure 8–8). The deeper the burn, the more severe it is. The extent of a burn, known as the percentage of the total body surface area (%TBSA), refers to the overall amount of the body that is burned. The greater the percentage burned, the more severe the burn, and the greater the chance for infection and death.

Occupational therapy is vital to the burn victim. Many people with severe full thickness or subdermal burns of the hands may lose their fingers and require adaptations to perform chosen activities. Additionally, as the

Superficial (First Degree)

Redness of affected area

Sensitive to touch

No blisters

Sunburn is an example of a superficial burn

Partial Thickness Burn (Second Degree)

Damage to the epidermis and the dermis

Reddened areas

Sensitive to touch

Blisters present

Full Thickness Burn (Third Degree)

Destruction of epidermal and dermal layers

Subcutaneous layer is destroyed

Figure 8-8. Classification of Burn Injuries

burns heal, the skin tissue is replaced by scar tissue that is not at all flexible and causes joints to contract, resulting in range of motion deficits and loss of function. The occupational therapist works to prevent joint contractures by ranging the joints, reducing scar tissue, and fabricating splints.

Cancer

Cancer is the uncontrolled growth of certain cells that invade the surrounding cells and frequently travel, or metastasize, to other places in the body. Cancer (Greek for "crab") is the second leading cause of death in the United States. The word "cancer" strikes fear into the hearts of most people, and rightfully so; around one million cases of cancer are diagnosed each year in the United States, and, of those, approximately half will die from it.

Cancer can be both painful and disfiguring to the patient. The treatment for cancer, although vastly improved over the years, remains invasive and often leaves the patient weak, sick, and disillusioned. Doctors who specialize in cancer, called oncologists, treat the disease with a variety of methods, including surgery, the removal of the cancer by cutting it out of the patient's body; radiation, the destruction of the tumor using radioactive materials; chemotherapy, the destruction of the tumor through the use of chemicals or drugs; and immune therapy, which uses antibodies to recognize and destroy the cancerous cells.

Occupational therapy intervention for the cancer patient will depend on the type of cancer and whether or not it is curable. For example, a woman with breast cancer who has recently undergone a right total radical mastectomy (that is, the complete removal of the right breast, as well as the surrounding muscles and lymph nodes) will require occupational therapy to help restore her strength and the range of motion in her right arm. However, because significant lymph tissue was also removed, she may require intervention for swelling in her arm and hand, known as lymphodema.

In addition to the physical problems caused by both the cancer and the mastectomy, other problems might exist—such as difficulty with bathing, hygiene, and dressing—that can be addressed by the occupational therapist. Following a mastectomy, many women also have problems with their self-image and many develop clinical depression. All of these issues can be addressed by the occupational therapist.

If the cancer is incurable and, therefore, terminal, occupational therapy is still indicated as a palliative (providing comfort and easing pain in lieu of a cure) in the client's final days. Occupational therapy can add life to days, rather than days to life, by helping these individuals continue to participate in everyday activities, no matter how mundane or trivial they may seem. Even though a person may be terminally ill, she has the right and the need to make a contribution to society, however small.

The occupational therapist sees the individual's role disruption in the foreground and the specific limitation, or disease process, in the background (Tigges and Marcil, 1988). Therefore, the diagnosis of a terminal illness should not stop the individual's need to engage in occupation. In fact, the need to engage in the occupational pursuit of one's choice may be one of the most important aspects of palliative care, second only to pain control.

Cardiovascular Disease

Cardiovascular, or heart, disease, is the leading cause of death in the United States. Although modern surgical techniques, technology, and medications have helped people with heart disease live longer, it remains a major problem. Contributing factors include our genes, our lifestyles, eating too much processed food, and not exercising enough.

Although the person with cardiac disease may live longer, he does not necessarily live better. This is, in part, where occupational therapy can help. As part of the cardiac rehabilitation team, the occupational therapist can help the client grade activities to reduce any unnecessary stress and slowly increase the amount of stress as the client's physical and cardiac conditions improve. The therapist can also educate the client in energy conservation techniques and the use of appropriate assistive devices to facilitate the pursuit of activities and occupations.

Carpal Tunnel Syndrome

Carpal tunnel syndrome (CTS) is probably the best-known example of a repetitive stress disorder; thus, I have given it its own section.

Carpal tunnel syndrome is a condition affecting one or both hands in which one of the three main nerves serving the hand, the median nerve, becomes entrapped by the bones of the wrist. These eight bones, called carpal bones, form a canal that allows the median nerve to enter the hand. Sometimes this canal becomes narrow and constricted, pressing on the median nerve and impairing its function. Think about crimping a garden hose and restricting the flow of water. This is essentially what happens when the carpal tunnel impinges the median nerve: the nerve transmissions are impaired. This results in numbness and pain on the thumb side of the hand and, if left untreated, can cause the hand muscles to waste away, or atrophy.

Chronic Obstructive Pulmonary Disease

Chronic obstructive pulmonary disease (COPD) is a blanket term that describes any chronic, progressive, and irreversible condition of the pulmonary system (lungs and accessory structures) that interferes with an individual's ability to breathe—that is, to exchange oxygen and carbon dioxide at the cellular (internal respiration) and pulmonary (external respiration) levels. Individuals with COPD frequently complain of fatigue and shortness of breath, and may also have a chronic cough.

Some of the causes of COPD are emphysema, chronic bronchitis, and asthma. The condition can be aggravated by cigarette smoke, pet dander, pollen, smog and air pollution, extremes of air temperature, and excessive odors (such as heavy perfumes). Many people with COPD are dependent on oxygen units and may require a manual or electric wheelchair for mobility.

The occupational therapist's role with the client with COPD is frequently one of education. The client must learn to avoid those environments that might aggravate the condition, and plan accordingly. The client must also be aware of safety issues, such as keeping open flames away from oxygen canisters (I cannot tell you how many times I have had to warn some of my clients about the dangers of smoking while using oxygen).

Perhaps the biggest goal of the occupational therapist working with the COPD client is that of energy conservation education. The client should not expend any unnecessary energy while performing daily activities. It may not seem like a big deal to a healthy individual, but standing at the bathroom sink to wash your hands and face, brush your teeth, shave, or put on makeup takes quite a bit of energy; your large leg and lower back muscles require a great deal of oxygen in order to function properly. If you were to sit on a high stool to perform these same activities, as people with COPD may need to do, you could still see yourself in the mirror, but you would use only a fraction of the oxygen for which other parts of your body are vying.

Chronic Pain Syndrome

Chronic pain syndrome (CPS) is a condition that is marked by ongoing, nearly constant pain from which a person is unable to find relief without medications or other means such as acupuncture, transcutaneous electrical nerve stimulation (TENS), biofeedback, or other forms of analgesia.

Chronic pain syndrome can result from any number of causes: injury, arthritis, fibromyalgia, and lupus, to name but a few. The individuals affected by chronic pain are essentially prisoners within their own bodies. Many of these people become addicted to medications or illegal drugs in an effort to escape the constant pain. The prolonged misery of this condition frequently leads to clinical depression, which makes the pain worse. Many people with CPS commit suicide in order to escape the misery. In fact, suicide is the leading cause of death among this population.

Pain is a little-understood phenomenon; chronic pain is even less understood. We need pain to tell us that something is wrong, but when pain will not go away, it consumes us and interferes with our daily lives.

Occupational therapy can help the person with chronic pain in a number of ways, including a focus on modalities (such as TENS or ultrasound), relaxation training, or diversional activities. Diversional activities are those activities that serve to take one's mind off of a problem—in this case, pain. One example of this type of activity was mentioned in Chapter 1, where I discussed the concept of flow, a state of total concentration on an activity to the exclusion of other stimuli, including pain.

Cerebrovascular Accident

A cerebrovascular accident (CVA), usually called a stroke, is commonly seen by occupational therapists and other rehabilitation personnel, perhaps more than any other diagnosis. A stroke is caused by an interruption of the blood supply to one or more parts of the brain. Because the brain controls all bodily functions, sensations, and intellect, the problems caused by a stroke are many and can range in severity from so slight as to be hardly noticeable, to paralysis or even death.

Most strokes are caused by a blood clot (thrombotic stroke) that gets caught in one of the many small blood vessels in and around the brain.

This clot blocks the flow of blood to a section of the brain, and that section dies. The symptoms of the stroke will depend on what part of the brain is affected and how badly.

A second type of stroke (hemorrhagic stroke) is caused when a blood vessel in the brain ruptures and blood spills into the brain, damaging the tissue. The more blood that invades the skull and displaces the brain tissue, the greater the damage and more severe the physical signs of stroke (such as speech problems, muscle weakness, and paralysis).

We typically picture someone with a stroke as having paralysis on one side of the body (hemiplegia), drooping facial muscles, and speech problems. Regardless of the physical symptoms, the individual will probably have difficulty performing the daily activities that most of us take for granted.

The occupational therapist working with a client who has suffered a stroke faces two main problem areas: helping to restore upper extremity muscle function and use, and helping the client learn how to function despite her disability.

The occupational therapist first evaluates the client's physical status in an effort to determine what physical problems might impair her function. Some degree of weakness or paralysis will typically exist on one side of the body. The occupational therapist works to normalize the muscle tone in the affected arm and hand. If there is too little muscle tone (weakness or flaccidity), the goal is to increase it; if there is too much muscle tone (spasticity), the goal is to reduce it. To normalize muscle tone, the occupational therapist and occupational therapy assistant use special neurophysiologic techniques that are beyond the scope of this book.

Whether or not muscle tone or other physical problems are remedied, the occupational therapist strives to help the client become as independent as possible. This can involve teaching the client how to perform tasks in a different way than she may be used to, and showing her how to use adaptive equipment to assist in the performance of an activity.

Coma

Coma is a complex and little-understood phenomenon. Coma is a state of profound unconsciousness in which the individual is unable to interact with his environment. Many people perceive a person in a coma as being deeply asleep—the difference being that a sleeping individual can be aroused with little or no difficulty, while the comatose individual cannot be aroused.

Different levels of coma exist, ranging from severe to mild, along with several coma rating scales. The two most common scales are the Glasgow Coma Scale and the Rancho Los Amigos Coma Scale (Figure 8–9). These

I. No Response

Patient appears to be in a deep sleep and is unresponsive to stimuli.

II. Generalized Response

Patient reacts inconsistently and non-purposefully to stimuli in a nonspecific manner. Reflexes are limited and often the same, regardless of stimuli presented.

III. Localized Response

Patient responses are specific but inconsistent, and are directly related to the type of stimulus presented, such as turning head toward a sound or focusing on a presented object. He may follow simple commands in an inconsistent and delayed manner.

IV. Confused-Agitated

Patient is in a heightened state of activity and is severely confused, disoriented, and unaware of present events. His behavior is frequently bizarre and inappropriate to his immediate environment. He is unable to perform self-care. If not physically disabled, he may perform automatic motor activities such as sitting, reaching, and walking as part of his agitated state, but not necessarily as a purposeful act.

V. Confused-Inappropriate, Non-Agitated

Patient appears alert and responds to simple commands. More complex commands, however, produce responses that are non-purposeful and random. The patient may show some agitated behavior, rather than internal confusion, in response to external stimuli. The patient is highly distractible and generally has difficulty learning new information. He can manage self-care activities with assistance. His memory is impaired, and verbalization is often inappropriate.

VI. Confused-Appropriate

Patient shows goal-directed behavior but relies on cueing for direction. He can relearn old skills, such as activities of daily living, but memory problems interfere with new learning. He has a beginning awareness of self and others.

VII. Automatic-Appropriate

Patient goes through daily routine automatically, but is robot-like with appropriate behavior and minimal confusion. He has shallow recall of activities and superficial awareness of, but lack of insight into, his condition. He requires at least minimal supervision because judgment, problem solving, and planning skills are impaired.

VIII. Purposeful-Appropriate

Patient is alert and oriented, and is able to recall and integrate past and recent events. He can learn new activities and continue in home and living skills, though deficits in stress tolerance, judgment, abstract reasoning, social, emotional, and intellectual capacities may persist.

Figure 8-9. Rancho Los Amigos Scale

scales are designed to ascertain the client's level of coma, based on things like visual tracking, vocalization, and level of confusion. Comatose clients frequently can ascend from the lower levels of coma to the higher levels of recovery.

A condition closely related to coma is known as persistent vegetative state (PVS). An individual in this condition appears to be awake and alert, but, in reality, her higher brain functions are nonexistent and she is actually functioning on the lower brain stem, which controls the vital basics of life such as breathing and heart rate. These individuals will continue to stay alive, as long as their hearts keep beating. However, one must always consider the difference between staying alive and living.

You may occasionally hear about people in this state at the center of legal battles over whether they are truly alive or, in fact, "brain dead." Sadly, these individuals no longer have the higher cerebral functioning that will allow them to think, feel, reason, or love again. In fact, many of these individuals are left senseless—unable to see, hear, smell, or feel things. They have no way to interact with their immediate environment. They have, in effect, ceased to be human. Although their hearts beat and their lungs exchange air, all of their biologic functions are on "autopilot." They must be catheterized for urine output, wear diapers for fecal output, be turned, bathed, and dressed, and have their arms and legs ranged to prevent contractures. There is no escape from this living death.

Complex Regional Pain Syndrome

Complex regional pain syndrome (CRPS), formerly known as reflex sympathetic dystrophy (RSD), is a chronic pain condition usually affecting the hands, arms, shoulders, feet, and legs. The pain, which can be intense and debilitating, is often disproportionate to the frequently mild injury that caused it. Although CRPS is not completely understood, it is thought to be neurovascular, involving blood vessels and the nerves that surround them.

Symptoms of CRPS include color and temperature changes of the skin of the affected body part, along with intense pain, swelling, and sweating. The pain caused by this condition can be incapacitating, and many sufferers contemplate or attempt suicide to escape its grip. This condition often occurs following a stroke and is sometimes referred to as shoulder-hand syndrome, because it tends to cause pain in both the affected arm and shoulder on the paralyzed side. This condition can further complicate the client's rehabilitation outcome.

When working with the client with CRPS, the occupational therapist seeks to improve the function of the affected arm and hand, increase range of motion, and decrease the pain and swelling associated with the condition. If the swelling can be reduced or eliminated, function will improve. To reduce swelling, the occupational therapist uses techniques such as active and passive range of motion, weight bearing on the affected arm and hand (known as stress loading), elevation, cold therapy, splinting, and compression garments.

Cumulative Trauma Disorders

An increase has occurred, in recent years, in the number of people who experience severe pain in various parts of the body that can be traced to an activity in which they frequently participate. These injuries, usually associated with the limbs, occur from constant repetitive movements and can result in what is sometimes called overuse syndrome or (more recently) cumulative trauma disorders. You may know these disorders by their common names, including tennis elbow, golfer's elbow, rotator cuff injuries, or runner's knee.

The occupational therapist may treat these injuries using modalities such as hot and cold packs, ultrasound, and splinting. However, the best way to protect against further problems is to evaluate the way the person performs a given activity and then help him correct it.

Diabetes

Diabetes mellitus (DM), often called sugar diabetes or "sugar," is a disease in which the body is unable to produce or properly utilize the hormone insulin, which is responsible for processing carbohydrates into the fuel the body needs to function. Due to the lack or absence of insulin, excessive glucose, or sugar, remains in the bloodstream—a condition known as **hyperglycemia.**

The most common form of diabetes is type 2 diabetes, the cause of which is a failure of the body to properly use the insufficient amount of insulin produced by the pancreas. Sometimes diabetes can be treated by diet, exercise, or oral medications; in this case, the diabetes is referred to as non-insulin dependent diabetes mellitus (NIDDM). The majority of diabetics, however, must inject themselves with insulin one or more times each day in order to keep their blood level in the normal range; this type of diabetes is referred to as insulin dependent diabetes mellitus (IDDM). These individuals monitor their blood sugar on a daily basis and adjust their insulin dosages accordingly. If too

Hyperglycemia (High Blood Sugar)

Extreme thirst (polydipsia)

Frequent urination (polyuria)

Dry skin with itching

Hunger

Blurred vision

Fatigue

Nausea

Hypoglycemia (Low Blood Sugar)

Sweating (diaphoresis)

Rapid heartbeat (tachycardia)

Anxiety

Irritability

Dizziness

Weakness, fatigue

Headache

Visual problems

Figure 8-10. Signs of Blood Sugar Imbalance

much insulin is used, the person may develop low blood sugar, or **hypoglycemia,** and possibly go into **insulin shock** or **insulin coma.** This is a medical emergency that can lead to death if not treated in a timely manner.

Although too little blood sugar can be deadly in the short term, too much blood sugar can have serious consequences in the long term, including high blood pressure, kidney problems, heart problems, blindness, amputations, and stroke (Figure 8–10). The diabetic ultimately sees the occupational therapist for one or more of these problems, and not necessarily for the diabetes.

A person with diabetes who has had a stroke and only has use of one hand will often require the assistance of an occupational therapist to show him how to test his blood sugar level using a special device known as a **glucometer.** He may also need training to help him to fill a syringe and inject himself with insulin. The ability to perform these tasks safely and independently can mean the difference between living at home or in a supervised residential setting.

Guillain-Barré Syndrome

Guillain-Barré syndrome (pronounced ghee-yan bah-ray) (GBS) is a disorder caused by the body's immune system that attacks the **peripheral nervous system** and results in muscle weakness and a tingling sensation in the limbs (**paresthesia**) (National Institute of Mental Health, 2004). The symptoms, which usually begin in the hands and feet, are thus described as a "glove and stocking distribution." The symptoms may then progress upward toward the trunk; for this reason, Guillain-Barré syndrome is often called **ascending paralysis.** The respiratory muscles can become paralyzed in severe cases and, if not treated immediately, may result in death. In the past, Guillain-Barré syndrome has been confused with other neurological disorders (Figure 8–11).

Franklin Delano Roosevelt, the four-term, 32nd president of the United States, had a physical disability for most of his adult life and throughout his entire presidency—a fact that he took great pains to keep hidden from the American public.

Roosevelt became gravely ill with fever and weakness at the age of 39, while vacationing in Canada. Days later, he was partially paralyzed and had severe pain in his legs. Polio was a great crippler of young people in the United States at the time, and it was assumed that Roosevelt had contracted it. Roosevelt used leg braces and a wheelchair for the rest of his life, until his death at the age of 65. Before he died, however, he opened a clinic for victims of polio in Warm Springs, Georgia (where he himself spent a great deal of time). Following his death in 1945, in part due to his condition, a great deal of research went into finding a cure for polio; the first polio vaccine was developed in the 1950s, and the disease that had disabled thousands of young Americans was eventually eradicated.

Ironically, recent speculation suggests that FDR never had polio to begin with. The fact that he first experienced symptoms at the relatively advanced age of 39, combined with reports of leg pain and other factors, has led researchers to believe that he instead suffered from Guillain-Barré syndrome.

Figure 8-11. President Franklin Delano Roosevelt was thought to have polio; however, recent evidence indicates that he may, in fact, have suffered from a completely different condition.

Guillain-Barré syndrome typically follows a cold or flu or, in some cases, a flu vaccination. An epidemic of swine flu in the United States during the 1970s led communities across the country to perform mass vaccinations. Many who received the vaccine developed GBS as a result, and quite a few died of respiratory complications. Normally, however, the condition is self limiting; with medical intervention and therapy, most people make a complete recovery within one year.

Occupational therapy for a person with Guillain-Barré syndrome may include strengthening exercises and fabricating hand splints to prevent contractures and deformities, as well as improving function. The therapist may also provide instruction in the use of assistive devices to make daily activities easier.

Head Injury

Closed head injury (CHI) occurs when damage is caused to the brain by blunt trauma to the head; circulation problems occur in the brain, such as an aneurysm or subdural hematoma; or the brain lacks oxygen (anoxia), caused by heart failure, drug overdose, infection (such as meningitis), or suffocation. A head injury differs from a stroke in the extent of the brain damage that occurs. While the damage caused by a stroke tends to be limited to a specific area of the brain, the damage caused by head trauma tends to be more widespread and diffuse, resulting in many more symptoms.

To get an idea of what happens in a head injury, imagine placing a rubber ball in a jar filled with water. When the jar is shaken, the ball will continue to move back and forth, bumping into the sides of the jar. This is essentially what happens to the brain in the event of a trauma, such as the head being forced into the windshield of a car. The brain, sitting in a pool of cerebrospinal fluid, is bounced back and forth against the skull; with each strike, brain damage occurs. Head injuries are much more complicated and, often, more devastating than strokes, which are more focused in their damage.

Those who sustain a serious head injury frequently will endure some degree of coma, and a percentage of them will enter a persistive vegetative state where they are unable to interact, in any meaningful way, with the outside world. Those in a coma can recover to some degree, in many instances, and occupational therapy can play a vital role in the rehabilitation process. Due to the complicated nature of head injury, it is important to note that occupational therapy is only one part of a total team effort between physicians, nurses, physical therapists, speech therapists, activities therapists, dieticians, and others.

Occupational therapy intervention for a person with a head injury may include active and passive exercises, splinting or casting of spastic limbs, muscle tone normalization, bed and wheelchair positioning, orientation to the environment, sensory training, and training in activities of daily living. The rehabilitation process for head injury is usually long term and intense in nature.

HIV/AIDS

The human immunodeficiency virus (HIV) is a relative newcomer to the world of virology and disease. Though believed to have been around since the 1950s, HIV did not make its presence known until the 1980s, at which time those who had been infected began to exhibit bizarre symptoms and exotic diseases rarely seen by physicians. Most of these individuals died without understanding what had killed them. By the mid-1980s this disease had a name: acquired immunodeficiency syndrome, or AIDS.

HIV was soon determined to be transmitted via sexual relations and contaminated blood. HIV belongs to a family of viruses known as retroviruses; that is, the virus can remain dormant and inactive within the host for a long period of time before any symptoms are noticed. Eventually, HIV integrates itself into the RNA of the host's immune cells and renders them useless—a kind of viral Trojan horse. Soon the immune cells begin to topple, one by one, and the infected host is unable to fight off even the simplest of infections.

Early on, a diagnosis of AIDS was essentially a death sentence. Today, however, researchers have developed many new drugs and therapies to help alleviate the symptoms of HIV/AIDS and to help those infected with the virus live longer, more productive lives. There is no cure for this infection as of yet, but it is no longer the death sentence it once was.

The best way to avoid exposure to HIV is by practicing safer sex—that is, limiting sexual partners and using proper barrier protection, such as latex condoms and dental dams, during sex. People may also practice universal precautions as outlined by the Centers for Disease Control (CDC) (Figure 8–12).

Because HIV infection can cause a wide range of symptoms, the role of occupational therapy is dependent upon the problems faced by the individual. Occupational therapists often focus on energy conservation, work simplification, assistive devices, and ADL training. Other areas may include strengthening, balance training, cognitive training, and vision training. Denton (1987) has outlined some suggested treatment phases and occupational therapy intervention strategies for the person with HIV/AIDS.

Universal precautions were established by the Centers for Disease Control (CDC, 1987) as a means of preventing the spread of HIV infection to and from health care workers. Universal precautions are important to follow at all times to prevent the spread of not only HIV but also diseases such as hepatitis, staphylococcal infections, influenza, and the common cold. You must treat all people with whom you come into contact as if they were infected with HIV or something similar and, at the same time, treat them as though you are infected as well. The idea is to prevent the spread of *anything* from one person to another.

The CDC recommends wearing gloves when touching bodily fluids such as blood, semen, vaginal secretions, and fluids from the brain, spinal cord, and heart. They place less emphasis on fluids such as feces, nasal secretions, saliva, sputum, urine, or vomit, because these are not methods of HIV transmission. I respectfully disagree with the CDC here, because other diseases can be transmitted through these fluids. My motto is: if it's wet, wear gloves. It's better to be safe than sorry.

Hand washing is another extremely important habit to develop. You should wash your hands frequently with soap and warm water. Hands should be washed at the start of the workday, before and after each client, before and after meals, after using the toilet, after coughing or sneezing in your hands, and before and after sex (this last one does not apply to work). **You must also wash your hands before and after using gloves.**

Figure 8-12. Universal precautions, as outlined by the Centers for Disease Control (CDC), should be employed at all times, regardless of with whom one is working.

Multiple Sclerosis

Multiple sclerosis (MS) is a disease of the central nervous system that can cause many physical problems. Multiple sclerosis affects about 300,000 people in the United States (women twice as often as men) and occurs between the ages of 15 and 50, giving it the reputation as the "crippler of young adults." Due to the many signs and symptoms of MS, it is sometimes also referred to as the "chameleon of other diseases." The actual cause of MS is unknown; however, it is widely thought to be an autoimmune disorder in which the body attacks its own nervous system.

Many of the nerve cells, or neurons, in our body are surrounded by a protective fatty insulation called **myelin,** which helps to conduct the nerve impulses more efficiently—much like the insulation on an electrical wire. This insulation is destroyed by MS, which causes a short circuit in the transmission of the nerve impulses. The myelin is replaced by scar tissue called **plaques** that further impede the transmission. These sclerotic plaques occur in multiple places throughout the nervous system—hence, the name "multiple" sclerosis.

These attacks, called **exacerbations,** occur periodically, causing symptoms such as weakness, visual problems, and spasticity. The symptoms may disappear just as suddenly as they appeared, in a process known as **remission.** For this reason, many people who go into remission think that they are cured, only to be disappointed when the next exacerbation occurs. As the disease progresses, the person becomes more and more disabled and unable to perform activities of daily living easily, if at all.

Any problem that affects one's limbs, vision, sensation, and coordination will obviously impact that person's ability to function. Fatigue is a major problem associated with MS; it is frequently all that the individual can do to muster up enough energy to participate in the simplest of activities. Occupational therapy has a great deal to offer these individuals, including muscle tone normalization, strengthening, splinting, ADL training, and energy conservation training. While addressing bathing and hygiene skills, the occupational therapist can inform the client that extremes of temperature (too hot or too cold) can impact her function, and care must therefore be taken when adjusting water temperature. If the client's environment is also too hot or too cold, her ability to function will be further impaired.

The occupational therapist working with a client with MS must always look ahead to the very real possibility that the client's condition will worsen in the future. The client should therefore be educated about possible adaptations or adaptive equipment that, although not needed in the present, may be necessary in the future.

Myasthenia Gravis

Myasthenia gravis (MG) is another autoimmune disease that causes generalized muscle weakness. It is not a disease of the muscles nor is it a disease of the nerves; the problem occurs at the spot where the nerves transmit signals to the muscle, the **neuromuscular junction.** Antibodies block or destroy the receptor sites for the neurotransmitter **acetylcholine,** and the muscle does not receive the signal to contract. This causes weakness in certain muscles. Think about how a radio works: the radio picks up the radio waves from the air by means of the antenna. If bad weather or an overpass interferes with the signal, you can't hear the radio, even though the signal is there and the radio is in working order. Instead, you just hear static.

The symptoms of myasthenia gravis are usually less noticeable when the individual is well rested, and they tend to get worse as the day progresses. Therefore, the occupational therapist can help the person with mild MG by instructing him to rest frequently throughout the day, as his muscles fatigue.

The person with MG may also have difficulty chewing and swallowing, due to muscle weakness. Working with the speech therapist, the occupational therapist can educate the individual on the proper positioning to prevent choking, cutting food into small pieces that are easier to swallow, and the use of assistive devices to facilitate the feeding process. As the disease progresses, the client gradually becomes more disabled and dependent upon others. The occupational therapist can help the client in most stages of the illness by adapting his environment to allow him some semblance of independence and control.

Orthopedic Injuries

Orthopedic injuries account for the majority of occupational therapy intervention, second only to cerebrovascular accidents in the physical rehabilitation practice arena. Orthopedics is the branch of medicine concerned with the prevention and correction of disorders of the locomotor system, including the bones, muscles, and joints (Mosby's Medical, Nursing, and Allied Health Dictionary, 1998). The term *orthopedic* literally means "straight child."

A great deal of orthopedic practice involves hip and knee joint replacements and surgical repair of broken bones. Following these surgical procedures, the client usually requires physical and occupational therapy.

The role of occupational therapy in orthopedics typically involves educating the client about different ways to perform daily activities. Following a total hip replacement (THR), for example, a client has restrictions on how far she can bend at the replaced hip. These restrictions can severely limit the activities that she can perform, including lower body dressing and bathing, and various household activities that require bending. The occupational therapist can teach the client alternative ways of performing these activities that do not involve bending, as well as how to use assistive devices to help facilitate the performance of the activities.

Osteoporosis

Osteoporosis is a condition marked by the loss of bone density, making bones porous and prone to fractures. Osteoporosis is most common in postmenopausal females, but it can also occur in people who are generally inactive and those with long-term steroid treatment or abuse. Osteoporosis is also one of the leading causes of broken hips; in fact, in many cases it is difficult to determine if a person's hip broke because she fell, or if she fell because her hip broke.

The occupational therapist can assist the client with osteoporosis by educating her on joint protection techniques, energy conservation techniques, work simplification techniques, and the use of adaptive equipment to facilitate daily activities. Fall prevention is another important area that should be addressed by the therapist; removing clutter and rearranging furniture (with the client's consent) can prevent trips, falls, and fractures.

Parkinson's Disease

Parkinson's disease (PD) is a progressive neurological condition that affects the part of the brain that produces the neurotransmitter **dopamine.** This results in a number of symptoms, including **resting tremors,** which are tremors that occur when the person is not actively or intentionally moving. The most common type of resting tremors seen in Parkinson's disease are called "pill rolling" tremors, in which the person appears to be rolling invisible pills between his thumb and index finger. Other symptoms of Parkinson's disease include muscle rigidity, difficulty initiating and stopping voluntary movement, and difficulty swallowing. As the disease progresses, the person eventually loses range of motion and the ability to walk. Many people with PD develop depression (possibly brought on by the lack of dopamine) and, eventually, dementia.

The most important goal of occupational therapy intervention with Parkinson's disease is to keep the client as mobile and active as possible. The effects of the disease can be held at bay by engaging the client in activities that promote gross motor functioning. Activities such as walking, dancing, and tai chi are excellent ways to help maintain function. Adaptive equipment may also be necessary to maintain independence and safety during activities such as eating, bathing, and dressing.

Post-Polio Syndrome

The neurological disease poliomyelitis (polio, or infantile paralysis) was perhaps the greatest public health threat that existed in the first half of the 20th century. The threat of this disease was so severe that parents would keep their children from public swimming pools in the summertime (when polio was thought to be most contagious) in an effort to keep them healthy.

The polio virus attacks the part of the central nervous system that is responsible for muscle movement, causing muscle weakness and paralysis, while sparing that part of the CNS responsible for sensation. Many victims of polio required the use of an iron lung to help them breathe because their respiratory muscles were paralyzed. This disease caused disability and sometimes death in tens of thousands of young people throughout the world.

Thanks to the development of the Salk vaccine in the 1950s, and the more user-friendly Sabin vaccine in the 1960s, polio has been virtually eliminated as a public health problem throughout most of the world. However, for many of the people who survived a bout with polio before the development of the vaccines, an unpleasant surprise awaited decades later.

"Post-polio syndrome (PPS) is a condition that can affect polio survivors anywhere from 10 to 40 years after recovery from an initial paralytic attack of the poliomyelitis virus" (National Institute of Neurological Disorders and Stroke, 2005). Between 25 and 50% of polio survivors are estimated to develop PPS.

The cause of PPS is thought to be the destruction of nerves that survived the initial polio infection, and its symptoms include fatigue, muscle weakness and atrophy, joint pain, and possible skeletal deformities as a result of muscular weakness and imbalance.

Occupational therapy intervention for people with PPS may include energy conservation, work simplification, and ergonomic training to help reduce the effects of fatigue. An exercise program to increase strength and endurance may also be indicated. Splints may be needed to reduce the possibility of joint contractures or to improve function during activities.

Spinal Cord Injury

Spinal cord injury (SCI) can result in partial or complete paralysis and sensory loss in part or most of the body. Most SCIs are the result of trauma to the back or neck from motor vehicle accidents, diving accidents (head first), and gun shot wounds (GSW), although some can occur from disease. Most victims of SCI are young males between the ages of 15 and 28, because they are more likely to engage in risky behaviors, sometimes under the influence of drugs and alcohol.

There are essentially two types of SCI: **quadriplegia,** or paralysis of both arms and both legs, and **paraplegia,** paralysis of both legs. If the injury occurs very high up on the neck, the accident victim will probably die instantly, because the brain stem controls vital bodily functions like breathing and heart rate. Some people with high SCIs manage to survive but require the use of a respirator to help them breathe. Most, if not all, people with SCIs have some form of bowel and bladder control problems.

Quadriplegics, in particular, have difficulty performing activities of daily living due to limited, if any, use of their arms and hands, as well as poor balance. Paraplegics have an easier time, because they can use their arms and hands and have better balance. People with SCIs must also be very aware of the condition of their skin, in order to prevent the development of pressure sores.

Occupational therapy is extremely important for people with spinal cord injuries. Quadriplegics must learn to use whatever upper-extremity functioning they have available to them. This typically requires extensive adaptive equipment and environmental adaptation to achieve the simplest of tasks, such as eating, turning the pages of a book, or changing the channel on a television set.

Advancements in technology have made life much easier for many quadriplegics. Computers have made it possible for those with limited mobility not only to write and communicate, but to operate environmental control systems that can open and close doors, open and close curtains, and turn lights, radios, and televisions on with the push of a button or key. Adaptive equipment, such as a dressing stick, reaching device, or button hook, can help the individual with a spinal cord injury to dress himself with greater, if not total, independence.

Splinting can help prevent joint contractures in people with spinal cord injuries and can reduce spasticity in joints, as well. For some quadriplegics, specifically those with C6–C7 injuries, splints (such as a **tenodesis** splint) can help improve what little function remains. The tenodesis splint is attached to the individual's wrist, so that when the person flexes his wrist, his fingers passively extend; when he actively extends his wrist, the tendons in his fingers shorten and allow him to pick up objects with his fingers.

Occupational therapists can also help people with spinal cord injuries in the area of driving. We are an extremely mobile society, and most of us drive cars. Modern technology has made it possible for those with spinal cord injuries to drive, as well. Hydraulic lifts and hand controls for acceleration and braking allow almost anyone with an SCI to access and drive a motor vehicle; frequently, the occupational therapist helps these individuals learn how to drive again.

Visual Impairments

Hundreds of thousands of people in the United States have some degree of visual impairment, ranging from near- or farsightedness to total blindness. Visual impairments can be present at birth (congenital) or acquired through an accident, disease, or old age (such as **cataracts, glaucoma,** and **macular degeneration**). Visual impairments can also occur following a stroke, head injury, HIV infection, poisoning, or diabetes.

Blindness occurs when one is unable to see anything out of one or both eyes. Total blindness is not as common as you might think; however, many people suffer from visual deficits that render them "legally blind"—that is, they are unsafe to operate motor vehicles and have difficulty with daily activities due to visual impairment. Those with a condition that seriously impairs their vision are said to have "low vision." Figure 8–13 demonstrates how people with various visual problems would read the word "balloon"; you can imagine the difficulty these individuals experience on a daily basis. Let us look at four of the main

BALLOON
Normal vision

LOON
Left hemianopia

BALL
Right hemianopia

LL   N
Left homonomous hemianopia

BA   OO
Right homonomous hemianopia

LLO
Bitemporal hemianopia (tunnel vision)

BA   ON
Macular degeneration

Figure 8-13. Visual problems come in all shapes and sizes.

causes of low vision: cataracts, glaucoma, macular degeneration, and diabetic retinopathy.

A cataract (from the Latin word for "waterfall") is the clouding of the lens of the eye, which results in decreased vision. This clouding is the result of the accumulation of proteins on the lens. When someone with cataracts looks at an object, she sees what looks like a halo surrounding it. To get an idea of what it is like to have cataracts, smear some Vaseline™ petroleum jelly on a pair of eyeglasses and try to read or watch television.

Although cataracts can be caused by many things, the most common cause is the aging process. Advances in medicine and technology allow the affected lens or lenses to be removed and replaced with a prosthetic lens.

Glaucoma is a buildup of pressure in the front portion of the eyeball caused by the inability of the eye to drain unneeded aqueous humor. Although there are often no symptoms of glaucoma, the buildup of intraocular pressure can cause gradual loss of peripheral vision, eye pain, and blurred vision. If left untreated—either by medication, surgery, or both—glaucoma can lead to blindness due to damage to the retina and optic nerve.

Macular degeneration is progressive damage to that part of the retina (the macula) responsible for the clearest vision. People with macular degeneration lose the ability to see things in their central visual field, as well as the ability to distinguish colors easily. These individuals must rely on their peripheral (side) vision, which can impair daily activities, including reading and watching television. There is no treatment for macular degeneration, although a certain type (the "wet" form) can be helped with laser surgery.

Diabetic retinopathy, one of the leading causes of blindness, results from long-standing or untreated diabetes mellitus. The retina is damaged over time by macular edema, hemorrhages, and the formation of new blood vessels in the retina.

For most of us, losing our vision—in part or in total—would bring about an abrupt change in our lifestyle. Imagine not being able to drive a car, watch television or a movie, read a book, or enjoy a sunset. It would be difficult to get around safely and easily, pick out clothes to wear, or cook a meal. Most of us take our vision for granted, yet there are tens of thousands of people in the United States with some degree of visual impairment beyond near- and farsightedness.

The occupational therapist or occupational therapy assistant can be of great help to individuals with visual impairments, by training them how to approach tasks and activities in a different manner and by using assistive devices to facilitate independence and safety. The occupational therapist can help the client make the most of her limited vision by demonstrating the proper use of lighting and magnifiers, color-coding items to make them easier to operate, and rearranging the living quarters for increased safety and user friendliness.

SUMMARY

This chapter has addressed the spectrum of illnesses and disorders that occupational therapists may treat in the course of their workday. These disorders have been divided into three main areas: developmental disabilities, mental health disorders, and physical disabilities. The disorders addressed in this chapter are some of the most common, but by no means all, of the possible disorders that a therapist might see in the course of a career.

References

American Psychiatric Association. (1994). *Diagnostic and statistical manual of mental disorders* (4th ed.). Washington, DC: Author.

Bonder, B. R. (1995). *Psychopathology and function.* Thorofare, NJ: Slack, Inc.

Brown, K., & Bradley, L. J. (2002). Reducing the stigma of mental illness. *Journal of Mental Health, 24*(1), 81–87.

Denton, R. (1986). An occupational therapy protocol for assessing infants and toddlers who fail to thrive. *American Journal of Occupational Therapy, 40*(5), 352–358.

Denton, R. (1987). AIDS: Guidelines for intervention. *American Journal of Occupational Therapy. 41*(7), 430.

Federal Register, volume 64, number 48. Code of Federal Regulations, Title 34, Section 300.7 [b] [9] (March 12, 1999).

Foti, D. (2005). Caring for the person of size. *OT Practice, 10*(2), 9–14.

March of Dimes. (2005). *Tay-Sachs disease.* Retrieved December 1, 2005 from http://www.marchofdimes.com/professionals/681_1227.asp

Mosby's medical, nursing, and allied health dictionary (5th ed.). (1998). St. Louis, MO: Mosby.

Muscular Dystrophy Association. (2005). *Myotonic muscular dystrophy.* Tucson, AZ: Muscular Dystrophy Association.

National Institute of Mental Health. (2004). *Autism spectrum disorders (pervasive developmental disorders).* Washington, DC: National Institute of Health.

National Institute of Neurological Disorders and Stroke. (2005). *Guillain-Barré syndrome information page*. Retrieved November 26, 2005 from http://www.ninds.nih.gov/disorders/gbs/gbs.htm

National Institute of Neurological Disorders and Stroke. (2005). *Post-polio syndrome information page*. Retrieved November 2, 2005 from http://www.ninds.nih.gov/disorders/post_polio/post_polio.htm

Poskey, G. A. (2005). Shaken baby syndrome: Prevention from an OT perspective. *OT Practice, 10*(22), 17–21.

Professional guide to diseases (8th ed.). (2005). Philadelphia, PA: Lippincott Williams & Wilkins.

Reed, K. L. (2001). *Quick reference to occupational therapy* (2nd ed.). Gaithersburg, MD: Aspen Publishers, Inc.

Satcher, D. (1999). *Mental health: A report from the surgeon general.* Washington, DC: Department of Health and Human Services.

Schindler, V. (2000). Occupational therapy in forensic psychiatry. In R. P. Flemming Cottrel (Ed.), *Proactive approaches in psychiatric occupational therapy* (pp. 319–325). Thorofare, NJ: Slack, Inc.

Seligman, M. E. P. (1975). *Helplessness: On depression, development, and death.* San Francisco, CA: Freeman.

The Sickle Cell Information Center. (2005). *Sickle cell disease.* Retrieved December 6, 2005 from http://www.scinfo.org/sicklept.htm

Stein, E., & Brown, J. D. (1991). Group therapy in a forensic setting. *Canadian Journal of Psychiatry, 36*, 718–722.

Tigges, K. N., & Marcil, W. M. (1988). *Terminal and life-threatening illness: An occupational behavior approach.* Thorofare, NJ: Slack, Inc.

CHAPTER 9

A Day in the Life of an Occupational Therapist

Chapter Goals

At the conclusion of this chapter, the reader will:

- Have a basic idea of the roles and responsibilities of occupational therapy personnel in a variety of treatment arenas.

INTRODUCTION

We all have different ways of learning new things. Some of us learn by reading about a subject. Some of us learn by listening to a lecturer or an audio program. Some of us learn by hands-on experience. The best approach to learning is the one that is most effective for you.

Sometimes, however, you can learn just by watching someone else do what you are hoping to learn about. Medical students know this approach as "see one, do one, teach one": the student first observes someone doing an appendectomy or two, then she does a few on her own, and, finally, she teaches the technique to another student.

To give you, the reader, a better idea of what an occupational therapist does in an average day, I would like to introduce you to a few of my colleagues: Sharon, who works in an outpatient clinic; Kent, who works in home health; Leigh Ann, who works for a school district; Anita, who works in a long-term care facility; and Carlos, who works in the psychiatric unit of a general hospital. After spending a day observing these therapists, you'll have a much better idea of how occupational therapy works.

Sharon: Outpatient Therapy

Sharon is a registered occupational therapist with three years of experience. She arrives at her clinic at 8:00 A.M. and prepares to see her first patient, Mrs. Aston, who is scheduled for 8:30 A.M. While waiting, Sharon reviews her schedule for the day and sees that she has a total of 12 clients scheduled. She reviews the treatment plans for each of her clients and begins to gather the equipment and materials she will need for each session.

With about 10 minutes to go before her first client arrives, Sharon writes a therapy summary report on a patient she discharged earlier in the week. This report will be sent to the patient's insurance company and is necessary for reimbursement for therapy services.

Mrs. Aston and her husband arrive on time, despite inclement weather. Mrs. Aston had a stroke several months ago, which left her dominant right side weak and her speech and vision impaired. After a short stay in the hospital, she spent six weeks at an inpatient rehabilitation center and then returned home, where she received physical, occupational, and speech therapies for an additional six weeks. She began outpatient therapy last week.

Sharon performed an initial occupational therapy evaluation and, based upon Mrs. Aston's desires, has focused on increasing her right upper-extremity strength, range of motion, and fine motor functioning. In order to achieve these goals, she will use weights to provide resistance to Mrs. Aston's muscles. As Mrs. Aston gradually gains strength, the weights will be increased to further strengthen her muscles. In combination with the graduated weight training, Sharon will help loosen up Mrs. Aston's muscles using passive range of motion (PROM) prior to beginning with the weights. This will also help prevent possible joint contractures, or shortening, and will ultimately allow her to regain increased strength and active range of motion (AROM).

Sharon is also focusing on Mrs. Aston's fine motor skills, in order to help her perform daily activities such as signing her name, using her computer, fastening her bra, buttoning her blouse, and tying her shoes. Sharon has Mrs. Aston practice touching, or opposing, her thumb to each of her fingers, and picking up and manipulating objects with her right hand, starting with larger items and gradually working down to very small ball bearings. She also has her work with elastic putty to increase the strength of the small muscles in her hand, which will also help to improve her coordination and dexterity. Sharon may occasionally use a nine-hole peg test to measure improvement in hand function, which will monitor whether her performance time decreases—an indicator of increased dexterity. She will also test her grip and pinch strength using a dynamometer and a pinch dynamometer.

Mrs. Aston's goals are to be able to take care of her house, cook meals for herself and her husband, and drive her car again. Her visual impairment could be problematic in each of these areas, but it is particularly dangerous in terms of driving her car. The stroke caused a condition known as right hemianopsia, or the ability to see out of only the right half of her right eye. Unless she compensates for this visual loss, she will not see anything on her right side. This visual impairment could cause Mrs. Aston to run off the side of the road or even hit a pedestrian walking along the side of the road. Sharon teaches Mrs. Aston to compensate by frequently turning her head to the right, in order to see anything that would normally appear in her peripheral vision. Sharon constantly reminds Mrs. Aston to do this, regardless of the activity she may be performing. Eventually, Sharon will perform a driving evaluation with Mrs. Aston to test her reflexes and reaction time, her ability to process stimuli, and her visual functions.

Kent: Home Health

While Sharon is working with Mrs. Aston, Kent is on his way to see his first client of the day. This will be an evaluation visit. The client, Mr. Samuels, has multiple sclerosis (MS), a neurological disease that affects muscle tone, strength, and coordination. Although he is not familiar with the neighborhood, Kent finds the apartment building and knocks on Mr. Samuel's door at 8:45 A.M. Mrs. Samuels answers the door and Kent introduces himself. Mrs. Samuels guides Kent to the bedroom, where Mr. Samuels is in bed.

Kent introduces himself to Mr. Samuels, and, after some small talk to make the couple feel comfortable, he explains what occupational therapy is and how it might help Mr. Samuels to be as independent as possible.

Mr. Samuels is a 38-year-old man who works as an accountant for a manufacturing company; he was diagnosed with MS five years ago. Until now, the MS has been a nuisance but has not interfered with his functioning. But this latest exacerbation, or worsening of symptoms, has left him extremely weak and fatigued, with slurred speech and double vision due to weak eye muscles that cause one of his eyes to turn in, making him appear cross-eyed.

During the course of the evaluation, Kent finds that Mr. Samuels has functional use of his dominant right hand and exhibits no sensory problems. His intellect is undisturbed, although he does demonstrate symptoms of depression. He expresses a strong desire to be independent in all aspects of self-care and wants to return to work as soon as possible.

When the physical evaluation is complete, Kent devises goals to be addressed, in collaboration with Mr. and Mrs. Samuels. By the end of the eight-week occupational therapy program, Mr. Samuels will: 1) increase his upper-extremity strength to fair plus (see Figure 7–6) by performing a daily home exercise program (HEP); 2) increase the strength of both his hands to 50 pounds, as tested by a dynamometer; 3) increase his bimanual fine motor skills to allow him to use a computer keyboard; 4) be independent in all aspects of dressing, bathing, and grooming, using assistive devices as necessary; and 5) demonstrate functional knowledge of energy conservation and work simplification techniques during activities. Kent additionally recommends that Mr. Samuels wear an eye patch over one eye to help eliminate the double vision.

Kent finishes up his evaluation and meeting with the Mr. and Mrs. Samuels. He plans to see Mr. Samuels three times a week for six weeks, and then only two times a week for the remaining two weeks (in home health jargon, this is written as 3w6, 2w2). He shares all of the information with Mr. and Mrs. Samuels and tells them that he will return two days later at 9:00 A.M.

Once he is back in his car, Kent finishes up the evaluation and treatment plan and signs his name. He does a lot of writing; each home health care visit must be thoroughly documented. He then picks up his cellular phone and calls his next client to tell her that he is on his way.

Leigh Ann: School-Based Therapy

As Kent is driving away from Mr. Samuels' apartment building, Leigh Ann is already seeing her fourth student of the morning. Leigh Ann is a certified occupational therapy assistant (COTA) with 10 years of experience, most of it in the public school system. As a school-based therapist, Leigh Ann focuses on the child's occupational role of student, which typically revolves around academic and vocational activities—skills that are the precursors to the worker role—and play activities as they may apply to the academic setting.

In the not-so-recent past, children with physical disabilities and learning problems were assigned to special educational facilities to better meet their needs. Today, however, these children are educated in the least restrictive environment possible, and most, if not all, have been integrated into public schools under an **inclusion** program. Due to the influx of special-needs children into the school system, most schools utilize occupational therapy services on a regular basis.

Leigh Ann is currently working with an eight-year-old second grader named Spencer who is having difficulty with his handwriting. Spencer is unable to hold a pencil well enough to write his name. Leigh Ann has tried numerous things to help him, including using a larger pencil, pencil grips, and building up the pencil with foam rubber tubing. These approaches have been mildly successful, but Spencer is still having problems.

Today, Leigh Ann has fabricated a special splint out of low-temperature thermoplastic material that allows Spencer to hold the pencil with little effort. He practices copying letters and plays "Connect the Dots" on the paper. He has a huge grin on his face because he is able to use the pencil without dropping it, and his lines are the straightest that he has ever made. Leigh Ann will let him practice this through next week and then follow up with him to see if this will work on a regular basis.

Leigh Ann sends Spencer back to his classroom, writes a therapy summary, and prepares to go to her next school. Leigh Ann is an **itinerant therapist;** that is, she travels to several different schools throughout her workweek. Her next school, where she will finish her workday, is about 20 minutes away.

Anita: Long-Term Care

Anita, another COTA with three years of experience, works in a long-term care facility (also called a nursing home). Most of the residents are elderly, but there are also some younger people present who require ongoing assistance for a number of reasons, including head injuries, strokes, HIV/AIDS, and spinal cord injuries.

Anita began her day at 7:00 A.M., helping residents perform their morning activities of daily living (ADLs). On this particular morning, she has four clients whom she is teaching to bathe, groom, and dress. She works closely with the certified nursing assistants (CNAs), who normally do things for the clients. She teaches the clients how to perform tasks in alternate ways or by using assistive devices. She instructs the CNAs in these same techniques and devices, but she also instructs them to only supervise and assist the residents; they are not to perform the tasks for them.

When she is finished with the morning ADL training, Anita makes her way to the dining room, where most of the residents are having breakfast. A number of residents have to be fed by staff members, due to physical impairments. Anita helps these residents feed themselves by modifying and improving their seating and, thus, their posture, and provides them with adaptive equipment to facilitate independent self-feeding. One of these residents is Mrs. Johnson.

Mrs. Johnson had a stroke that resulted in weakness on her left side but also caused tremors in her dominant right side. These tremors make it almost impossible for her to bring food from her plate to her mouth without spilling it. Severe arthritis also makes it difficult for her to hold onto eating utensils. The entire dining process is difficult, messy, and frustrating for Mrs. Johnson, and she has given up and allows staff to feed her, although she doesn't really like it because it makes her "feel like a baby."

Anita begins with Mrs. Johnson's positioning in her chair. Anita pulls Mrs. Johnson further up in the chair, pushes the chair closer to the table, and places her feet flat on the floor. This seemingly simple maneuver helps Mrs. Johnson sit up straight and moves her closer to her food, reducing the distance from her plate to her mouth. This will also improve her ability to swallow and will reduce the possibility of choking or aspirating (inhaling) her food. Anita then places a lumbar support cushion behind Mrs. Johnson's back to provide support and comfort to her lower back.

Next, Anita provides Mrs. Johnson with a nonslip pad to place under her plate, to prevent it from sliding around on the table. She also attaches a plate guard to the plate, which will prevent food from falling off and make it easier for Mrs. Johnson to get food onto her eating utensils. Anita gives Mrs. Johnson a large-handled fork, which is easier for her to hold (due to her arthritis) and puts less strain on her joints. Inside the handle of the fork are lead weights totaling approximately one pound. This weight helps to decrease the intention tremors that Mrs. Johnson experiences when she attempts to bring the fork to her mouth. Finally, for additional stability, Anita has Mrs. Johnson place her right elbow on the tabletop in order to increase her control of the fork while eating.

Now that Mrs. Johnson is positioned properly and provided with the appropriate adaptive equipment, Anita observes her as she attempts to feed herself. Anita gently encourages her and provides occasional physical assistance as needed. Mrs. Johnson smiles broadly as she brings her scrambled eggs to her mouth without spilling. Anita praises her and encourages her to continue. She then instructs the assisting CNA to let Mrs. Johnson do as much for herself as possible. Anita has not only helped to increase Mrs. Johnson's independence, she has also freed up a nursing assistant who is now able to help another resident.

Carlos: Mental Health

Carlos begins his day by running an organizational skills development group for men with alcoholism. Five members belong to the group, and Carlos acts as the facilitator. Most of the men have very poor organizational skills, which lead to daily disorganization and frustration and, ultimately, contribute to their alcoholism. All of the group members are currently unemployed, partly due to their lack of organization and partly as a result of their drinking.

Most of the group members are having difficulty accepting the fact that they are in a mental health facility in the first place. Three of the five men are there as a result of alcohol-related traffic violations. Most alcoholics deny that they have a problem in the first place, as Carlos is quite aware. If this denial can be broken down, the alcoholic can begin to help himself to a better life.

The first step in organizing the group involves getting all of the members to the meeting room by 8:30 A.M. This turns out to be a task in itself. Carlos must go to each group member's room and make sure that he is up and dressed. By 8:35 A.M., all of the members are finally present, albeit grudgingly. Carlos, realizing that he has his work cut out for him, introduces himself to the group, and has each of the members do the same.

By the time all of the introductions have been made, and Carlos has explained the purpose of the group and answered questions from the members, it is 9:30 A.M. Carlos wraps up the meeting and the group agrees to meet the next morning, promptly at 8:30 A.M.

Sharon

Back at the outpatient clinic, Sharon prepares for her session with Linda, an office manager who has developed **carpal tunnel syndrome (CTS),** caused by compression of the medial nerve by the wrist bones in her right hand. The pain and numbness in her hand make it very difficult for Linda to perform most aspects of her job.

Sharon begins the session by using **ultrasound** on Linda's right wrist. This treatment helps relieve the pain of the CTS by penetrating deep into the soft-tissue with high-frequency sound waves that produce heat. Ultrasound treatment is usually very successful in relieving the pain of CTS.

During the 10-minute ultrasound treatment, Sharon talks with Linda about possible ways she can perform her job skills that will decrease the chances of aggravating her CTS and making it even worse—a situation that might require surgery to correct. Because Linda spends a great deal of time using her computer, Sharon suggests that she consider using a commercially available wrist rest to provide support to her wrists while typing. Indeed, most cases of carpal tunnel syndrome are caused by excessive keyboarding, due to the way the typist's wrists are positioned for long periods of time. Carpal tunnel syndrome is one of many disorders caused by a **repetitive stress injury,** an injury that results from performing the same motion over and over again. Sharon explains that, through proper positioning and support of her wrists, Linda can decrease the pain in her right wrist and prevent her left wrist from suffering the same fate.

Following the ultrasound treatment, Sharon measures Linda's right hand and, using a low-temperature thermoplastic, fabricates a wrist support splint that will immobilize Linda's wrist to further decrease the pain and swelling of the carpal tunnel syndrome. Linda watches in amazement as Sharon heats up the hard plastic in a pan of warm water, removes it, and applies the now warm, soft, and pliable material to her wrist and hand. Within minutes, the plastic hardens into a firm, form-fitting splint.

Sharon enjoys this type of work. In addition to being a registered occupational therapist, she has received specialty training as a certified hand therapist (CHT). Once the splint is formed and hardened, Sharon makes straps for it and then teaches Linda how to apply and remove it, how long to wear it, how to spot signs of pressure areas, and how to clean and maintain the splint.

Kent

By 11:00 A.M., Kent is pulling up to his next client's house in a subsidized housing development. Kent is always amazed at the variety of people he sees in the home health care arena. On any given day, he will see clients who live in million-dollar waterfront houses and clients who live in neighborhoods like this one. He has worked in rural houses with no indoor plumbing, as well as in trailers, mobile homes, and hotel rooms. He even saw one client who lived on a boat in a marina.

His current client, Jerome, is a 19-year-old man who was shot in the chest while walking home from a party. The injury has severed his spinal cord and left him a **paraplegic,** or unable to move from his chest down. Jerome used to love to play basketball, but now he spends his days in bed, watching television and smoking cigarettes and marijuana. Jerome is extremely bitter about his injury and subsequent disability. Kent finds it difficult to motivate him to do anything.

Kent knocks on the door and Jerome's girlfriend, Tanyaa, lets him in. Jerome is in bed, watching television as usual. Kent greets Jerome and encourages him to sit up on the edge of the bed. After a while, Jerome agrees. Kent then encourages him to transfer into his wheelchair. Today is a good day; Jerome agrees, and Kent supervises him as he transfers from bed to wheelchair using a **transfer board,** a smoothly sanded and shellacked board, about 22 inches long, used to help perform safe transfers.

Now that he is sitting up in his wheelchair, Kent encourages Jerome to get dressed in street clothes. Jerome balks, stating that there isn't any sense in that because he's not going outside. Kent makes a deal with Jerome: he won't press the dressing issue if Jerome agrees to try some assistive devices to help him put on his pants, socks, and shoes. Jerome agrees to this and allows Kent to show him how to use a **sock aid,** a **dressing stick,** and a **long shoehorn.**

Once Kent shows him how to use these devices, and he tries them himself, Jerome begins to laugh and delights in playing with his new "toys." Before he realizes it, Jerome has put on his pants, socks, and shoes by himself. Kent understands that this has been a more successful session than he originally anticipated and decides not to push his luck any further. He makes arrangements to return in two days, and Jerome agrees to stay out of bed "for a while." Upon hearing this bit of good news, Kent reviews the transfer process with Jerome and Tanyaa and has her practice the transfer twice until both she and Jerome feel comfortable with her expertise. At that point, Kent says his good-byes and heads for his next appointment.

Leigh Ann

After lunch, Leigh Ann goes to a classroom and picks up two students, Brooke and Aiden, both of whom have **sensory integration** problems that interfere with their schoolwork as well as other activities of daily living. Leigh Ann brings them to the therapy room, which is filled with things that the children find fun and look forward to, such as giant balls on which they can sit and lay, a large Tumbleform® container filled with multicolored plastic balls, nets hanging from the ceiling, skateboards, and various mats, rolls, and wedges.

Leigh Ann starts the session using the nets. She places Brooke and Aiden in separate nets, because Aiden tends to be rambunctious and hyper. Leigh Ann pushes him in the net slowly, to help calm him down and prepare him for the upcoming activities. Brooke, on the other hand, tends to react slowly to stimuli; therefore, Leigh Ann rocks her quickly, in order to stimulate her prior to engaging in activities.

Once both children have finished with the nets, Leigh Ann engages them in a puzzle to help them focus and concentrate effectively on an activity that will be helpful in classroom learning and participation skills. Brooke tends to do better than Aiden, who is easily distracted. Leigh Ann gives him frequent verbal cues to attend to his task.

Toward the end of the session, Leigh Ann allows both children to play in the plastic ball container. This is what they really want to do, and Leigh Ann uses it as a reward for good behavior and participation in therapy. After 5 to 10 minutes of play, it's time to return to the classroom.

Anita

Meanwhile, Anita has continued to see residents in the occupational therapy clinic since breakfast. Currently, she is running a **gross motor** group for some of the residents with Parkinson's disease. These residents need to maintain their mobility and balance, and this biweekly group is one way for them to achieve this goal. Anita begins the group with a marching-in-place activity set to band leader John Philip Sousa's music. This music is not only familiar to the residents, it helps them to perform the movements more easily by providing a cadence to which they can easily move. The music also makes the activity fun.

After performing some upper-body stretching exercises, Anita engages the group in a game of "free-for-all" catch using an oversized rubber ball. The idea of this game is not to catch the ball but to get rid of it in any way possible. The participants can push it away with their arms and hands or kick it away with their feet and legs. This may seem childish and unimportant, but it is very important to these individuals; Parkinsonians have a difficult time initiating movements, and this game helps them perform automatic gross motor movements more readily while having fun at the same time. The game will help them to move more easily, maintain their balance, prevent falls, and make their daily living skills safer.

Carlos

At 11:00 A.M., Carlos meets with a group of three teenaged boys who have anger management problems. Each of these boys has been in trouble in school, and with the police, prior to admission to the hospital.

Carlos has chosen to use clay activities with this group. He has found that allowing the boys to get their hands dirty and knead the clay provides them with a constructive avenue for expressing their anger. The act of wedging the clay has been very helpful to the boys. Wedging clay involves taking very watery clay and throwing it against a wedging board over and over again, until the excess water has been removed and the clay can be molded. This group really enjoys wedging the clay, and they have had a number of good-natured competitions in recent days.

Although this may appear to be fun and games, the process is an educational one. Angry outbursts have occurred on more than one occasion, and more than one promising sculpture has been reduced to a pancake-shaped blob on the floor of the occupational therapy room. It is Carlos's job, at this point, to help the boys understand the results of their outbursts and see how their actions can affect themselves and others.

Sharon

Back at the outpatient clinic, Sharon has just started working with Henry, who was injured on his job as a dock worker and is now receiving work hardening therapy through his workers' compensation insurance. Henry injured his back by picking up a box that was heavier than he thought, and he has been unable to work for the past four weeks as a result.

Sharon has been working with Henry for the past two weeks on work hardening. She has taught him how to properly pick up objects of various weights by bending at his knees (rather than at his back), keeping his back straight at all times, and lifting the object more effectively. In essence, she is teaching him to work smarter, not harder.

Sharon must watch Henry carefully and document the therapy process and his progress very meticulously for workers' compensation insurance. She has seen her fair share of malingerers in her role as a work-hardening therapist. A malingerer is someone who feigns an illness or injury for the purpose of collecting workers' compensation, when, in fact, he is perfectly capable of performing his job. Sharon has frequently been called to serve as an expert witness in court cases involving workers' compensation and other insurance issues regarding an individual's ability to work.

In addition to teaching Henry about proper lifting techniques and body mechanics, Sharon has also instructed him in the use of a back support belt while performing lifting and heavy labor. Although research has shown that these belts do not actually prevent back injuries, they do serve to remind the wearer to keep his back straight while lifting.

Following this session, Sharon carefully documents Henry's progress and anticipates that he should be able to return to work within two to three weeks. She ends her workday by finishing off the day's documentation, and she glances at her calendar to review the next day's schedule.

Kent

As his workday nears its end, Kent pulls into the driveway of his seventh and final patient. This palatial house sits on waterfront property and has a beautiful view of the bay. Kent rings the doorbell and is greeted by Marjorie, a woman in her 40s, who guides him to the den where her mother, Mrs. Cooper, is watching television. Mrs. Cooper is a 70-year-old woman who recently broke her right hip as a result of a fall in her garden. Mrs. Cooper has a history of osteoporosis, a disease that causes bones to become brittle and easily broken.

Kent greets Mrs. Cooper, and they set to work. The first order of business is to help Mrs. Cooper safely stand up from her chair with little or no help. Kent shows her how to correctly position herself on the chair in order to use proper body mechanics to stand up. This involves Mrs. Cooper positioning herself at the edge of the seat, leaning forward over her body's **center of gravity,** and lifting her body into an upright position. Because Mrs. Cooper's favorite armchair is so low, this proves to be a difficult task. Kent then places an extra pillow on the chair to raise the sitting height; this makes the process easier. Kent explains to Mrs. Cooper and Marjorie that it is easier for his client to stand up if she is sitting in a higher chair. Although the cushion seems to work well, Kent explains that he can adapt the armchair even more by building a platform to make it higher, or Mrs. Cooper can consider purchasing an electric lift chair that would literally raise her to a standing position with the push of a button. Mrs. Cooper tells Kent that she will think about it and let him know on his next visit.

Kent then shows Mrs. Cooper some adaptive equipment to help her dress herself independently. Due to her hip fracture, Mrs. Cooper is unable to bend very far and, therefore, needs assistance to dress her lower body. Kent shows her how to use a dressing stick, sock aid, and long shoehorn. He first demonstrates how each device works and then lets her try them for herself.

Mrs. Cooper initially has some trouble manipulating the devices, but, after a few attempts, she masters each one. She starts to smile and then begins to laugh as her socks easily slide onto each foot. "I don't need your help anymore," she says to her daughter triumphantly. Kent then shows Mrs. Cooper some elastic shoelaces that she can use so she will not have to bend over to tie her shoes. Mrs. Cooper is beaming with pride in her accomplishments.

Kent tells Mrs. Cooper and Marjorie that he will return at the same time in two days for their next session, and then departs. He will stop at the office on his way home to finish his notes from the day and to turn in all of his paperwork. It has been a long day, but Kent is feeling great.

Leigh Ann

Leigh Ann has finished with all of her students by 3:00 P.M. and is now sitting down to help plan an Individualized Educational Program (IEP) for Eric, a new student at the school, who has attention-deficit hyperactivity disorder (ADHD). The IEP is a requirement of the Individuals with Disabilities Education Act (IDEA) for school-aged children with disabilities.

Present at the IEP meeting are Eric's teacher, his parents, and Eric himself. A physical therapist and a speech pathologist are also present, in addition to Leigh Ann and her immediate occupational therapy supervisor, Tony.

The meeting begins with Yvonne, the special education teacher, introducing herself and the other members present. She asks Eric and his parents to talk about Eric's strengths and weaknesses, as well as their expectations of the school district. This will give the group an idea of what direction the IEP meeting should take.

Leigh Ann and Tony listen to the conversation and ask questions from time to time regarding Eric's occupational therapy needs. The physical therapist and speech pathologist also ask questions regarding the possible needs of their professional involvement.

By the end of the 90-minute meeting, the IEP has been hammered out with input from all parties, including Eric and his parents. Leigh Ann will focus on sensory integrative issues to help Eric become better able to concentrate on tasks, as well as on Eric's handwriting skills.

Most afternoons at this time, Leigh Ann would be writing notes, planning the next day's activities, or meeting with Tony for a supervisory session. Before leaving the school, she glances at her schedule for the next day and then heads for her car.

Anita

After lunch, Anita begins to see residents in the occupational therapy room. Rather than have residents sit and lift weights or stack cones on a table, Anita tries to engage her clients in meaningful activities that can meet their physical, cognitive, psychological, and social needs.

Today, Anita has a small group of residents baking cookies. She has divided up the task into different components that serve the needs of specific residents. Mrs. Lincoln's job is to figure out which ingredients are required by the recipe and, using the energy conservation techniques that Anita taught her in a previous session, gather them all together.

Ms. Davis has been given the task of opening the various containers and packages in which the ingredients are held. A recent stroke has left her with the use of only her right arm, so she must perform each task using various adaptations, including nonslip Dycem® pads, an electric jar opener, and scissors. This task also requires Ms. Davis to attend to her left side in order to compensate for her left hemianopsia. Anita supervises Ms. Davis and lets her know if she misses anything.

Mrs. Nixon compiles all of the ingredients and mixes them together. This helps her sequence the steps required, and it increases the range of motion and strength in her right arm. Because Mrs. Nixon's grip strength is poor, Anita has adapted the wooden mixing spoon with neoprene foam to make it easier for her to grasp.

Mrs. Lincoln now takes the cookie dough, kneads it, rolls it flat with a rolling pin, and uses cookie cutters to shape the various cookies. These seemingly insignificant activities are helping to increase the strength in both of her hands, due to the resistance of the cookie dough.

Mrs. Capone will be the baker. She walks over to the oven, sets the baking temperature, and turns it on. It will be her job to put the cookies into the oven and remove them when they are finished. She doesn't realize it, but she is increasing her upper extremity range of motion and strength, as well as her endurance, during this task.

Mr. Rubenstein has announced that he will be the official cookie taster. This draws a laugh from the group. He initially wanted no part of the cookie preparation process but agreed to do the dishes when everything was done. His female peers readily agree to this arrangement.

Carlos

By the end of his workday, Carlos is wiped out. He has one more group to run, and he has saved this one for the end of the day to help himself as much as his clients. This last group is designed to help promote teamwork and interdependence among several emotionally disturbed teenagers.

Carlos has chosen a game of basketball for the group. This activity will teach them how to cooperate with each other while simultaneously allowing them to expend pent-up energy. For Carlos, however, the act of engaging in this activity himself will allow him to recharge his own batteries after a long, emotionally draining day.

Carlos often wonders if what he does is really work. It seems to him that much of what he does is just common sense, yet the people with whom he works have so much trouble with the simplest aspects of daily life: time management, organizational skills, relaxation, and basic life skills. Many of their problems, he realizes, are caused by an imbalance in their occupational performance areas of work, self-care, play and leisure, rest, and sleep. This is what he is here to do, to help these people find that balance and function adequately within society.

SUMMARY

This chapter has presented some vignettes to help give you a general idea of what occupational therapy is and how it works. These are general scenarios and do not represent the entire profession. This chapter is designed to give you a better idea of the occupational therapy process, as well as the varied practice areas in which occupational therapy personnel frequently work.

The overall purpose of this book has been to give you an understanding and appreciation of the art and science of occupational therapy. I have tried to make this an informative and entertaining process, and I sincerely hope that you have learned something about the profession that has shaped so much of my own life.

Frequently Asked Questions about Occupational Therapy

1. **What is occupational therapy?** Occupational therapy helps people who have been disabled by physical, developmental, and psychosocial diseases or impairments participate in their occupational roles of choice in the areas of self-care, work, and play and leisure. Occupational therapy involves the use of functional, meaningful activities to achieve the client's goals. Frequently the activity or the immediate environment must be modified or adapted to enable the client to participate.

2. **What does an occupational therapist do?** The ultimate goal of occupational therapy is to allow the client to participate in chosen occupational roles of work, self-care, and play and leisure. The therapist may perform evaluations in order to determine the client's strengths and weaknesses and, based on this evaluation, will develop a treatment plan to help the client achieve his desired occupational roles. The therapist may utilize any number of methods to meet the client's goals, including exercise, splinting, adaptive equipment/assistive devices/assistive technology, sensory integration, group activities, work hardening, and cognitive retraining, to name but a few.

3. **How much schooling is required to become an occupational therapist?** Beginning in 2007, all entry-level occupational therapists, registered (OTRs) will require a master's degree in occupational therapy (MOT); this will require a total of five years of college. An occupational therapy assistant (OTA) can expect to go to school for two years and graduate with an associate's degree.

4. **Do occupational therapists need to be licensed?** Most states and U.S. territories require occupational therapists and occupational therapy assistants to be regulated in some fashion, such as through licensing, certification, or trademark law. However, this is not universal, and these requirements vary from state to state. Some states also require regulation for OTRs but not for certified occupational therapy assistants (COTAs). You should check with your state to obtain information on the standing regulations.

5. **What is the difference between occupational therapy and physical therapy?** Physical therapy deals specifically with physical disorders of the body, and is aimed at restoring the use of weakened muscles, restoring normal movement, and decreasing pain. Occupational therapy is aimed at promoting an individual's independence in occupational role performance in the areas of self-care, work, and play and leisure. Although the two professions sometimes overlap in their techniques and approaches, they are two distinct fields that frequently augment and complement each other.

6. **How much does an occupational therapist earn?** Entry-level occupational therapists earn an average of $50,000 per year, and occupational therapy assistants earn an average of $34,000 per year. These figures will vary throughout the United States.

7. **What is the difference between an OTR and a COTA?** The primary difference between the two is the amount of required education. An entry-level occupational therapist with a basic master's degree will complete a total of five years of college, while the occupational therapy assistant can expect to attend college for two years in order to receive an associate's degree. An OTR can conduct complete occupational therapy evaluations, write treatment plans, and carry out treatment sessions. The COTA can assist the OTR in some aspects of the evaluation process and treatment planning, as well as provide direct patient treatment under the supervision of an occupational therapist. Although the two may appear to be very similar in their job descriptions, the COTA requires ongoing OTR supervision. The OTR, on the other hand, has more autonomy and usually does more paperwork as a result.

8. **Where do occupational therapists work?** The vast majority of occupational therapists and occupational therapy assistants work in hospitals, rehabilitation centers, long-term care facilities, and transitional care centers. Other areas of practice include home health, hospice, school systems, private practices, and psychiatric facilities. You may find an occupational therapist anywhere people are having problems achieving their occupational roles.

9. **How do I find an occupational therapy school?** Occupational therapy assistant and entry-level programs are available is most U.S. states and in Puerto Rico. The easiest way to find an occupational therapy program is by going to the American Occupational Therapy Association's Web site at http://www.aota.org, clicking on "Students," and choosing between OT or OTA programs.

10. **How many occupational therapists does it take to change a light bulb?** Actually, occupational therapists do not change light bulbs. They teach people how to do it themselves, sometimes using assistive devices.

11. **Can a COTA become an OTR?** Yes; there are two ways that this can be accomplished. First, the individual can build upon her associate's degree by taking additional courses, including any prerequisites a school may require. The second way is by attending a weekend program. These programs, which are few and far between, involve attending intensive weekend classes held approximately every few weeks. In addition to requiring a great deal of self-discipline, these programs, for many students, also require a great deal of travel and lodging expenses.

12. **What types of people need occupational therapy?** Any person who has difficulty with, or an inability to carry out, the occupational roles of work, self-care, and play and leisure can benefit from occupational therapy. This includes people with physical impairments such as arthritis, stroke, head trauma, orthopedic problems, and cardiac problems. It also includes children and adults with developmental disabilities (such as cerebral palsy), those with psychiatric problems, and others.

13. **Is there a national organization for occupational therapists?** The national organization for occupational therapists is the American Occupational Therapy Association, Inc., 4720 Montgomery Lane, P.O. Box 31220, Bethesda, MD 20824-1220. Each state also has its own association.

14. **Do other countries have occupational therapists?** According to the World Federation of Occupational Therapists (WFOT), there are 65 countries worldwide with members, associate members, or contributing members.

15. **Who pays for occupational therapy services?** The U.S. government, by way of Medicare, is the largest spender on occupational therapy services. Other sources of reimbursement include Medicaid, private insurance companies, workers' compensation, and private pay.

16. **What is the employment outlook for occupational therapists?** Occupational therapy continues to be one of the fastest growing professions today. The Bureau of Labor Statistics expects the need for occupational therapy personnel to grow steadily through the year 2012 and beyond. This is particularly true as the "baby boomers" grow older and require more occupational therapy services.

17. **Are there different kinds of occupational therapists?** All occupational therapists receive the same basic education. Most practicing therapists specialize in certain areas, such as psychosocial practice, hand therapy, physical disabilities, work hardening, pediatrics, and school-based practice.

18. **With what other professions do occupational therapists work?** The occupational therapist and occupational therapy assistant work in tandem with numerous other professionals, including physicians, nurses, physical therapists, speech and language pathologists, recreational therapists, activities therapists, and teachers.

19. **What is the difference between occupational therapy and therapeutic recreation?** Although occupational therapy and therapeutic recreation both grew from the same historic roots and sometimes seem to be very similar, major differences exist between the two professions. While occupational therapy focuses on work, self-care, and play and leisure, it has not focused much attention on the play and leisure aspect in recent years. With the exception of using play in their work with children, occupational therapists have primarily turned that area over to recreational therapists. One major difference between the two professions, however, is salary. While a COTA can expect to earn approximately $34,000 per year and an entry-level OTR can expect to earn around $50,000 per year, a recreational therapist can expect to earn only about $28,000 per year.

20. **What is the difference between occupational therapy and activities therapy?** This is really a matter of semantics. An activities therapist is actually a recreational therapist. However, a recreational therapist typically possesses a bachelor's degree and has been certified through the National Council for Therapeutic Recreation Certification (NCTRC). Activities therapy is primarily designed to keep people busily involved in activities that may or may not have a therapeutic goal other than just being fun for the client. A COTA can function as an activities therapist and does not require OTR supervision in this role.

APPENDIX B

Important Contact Information for Occupational Therapy

American Occupational Therapy Association, Inc. (AOTA)
4720 Montgomery Lane
Bethesda, MD 20824-3425
800-729-2682 (800-SAY-AOTA)
http://www.aota.org

National Board for Certification in Occupational Therapy (NBCOT)
The Eugene B. Casey Building
800 South Frederick Avenue
Suite 200
Gaithersburg, MD 20877-4150
301-990-7979
http://www.nbcot.org

Accreditation Council for Occupational Therapy Education (ACOTE)
ACOTE
c/o AOTA Accreditation Department
P.O. Box 31220
Bethesda, MD 20824-1220
301-652-2682
accred@aota.org

World Federation of Occupational Therapists (WFOT)
c/o WFOT Secretariat
P.O. Box 30
Forrestfield
Western Australia 6058
61 8 9453 9746
wfot@multiline.com.au

To locate state occupational therapy organizations, I would suggest that you Google™ "occupational therapy" and the state of your choice. Just about every state occupational therapy organization has its own Web site.

APPENDIX C

Recommended Further Readings on Occupational Therapy

Bing, R. K. (1981). Occupational therapy revisited: A paraphrastic journey. *American Journal of Occupational Therapy, 35*, 499–518.

Meyer, A. (1922). The philosophy of occupational therapy. *Archives of Occupational Therapy, 1*, 1–10.

Peloquin, S. M. (1989). Sustaining the art of practice in occupational therapy. *American Journal of Occupational Therapy, 43*, 219–226.

Reed, K. L. (1986). Tools of practice: Heritage or baggage? *American Journal of Occupational Therapy, 40*, 597–605.

Reed, K. L., & Sanderson, S. N. (1999). *Concepts of occupational therapy* (4th ed.). Philadelphia, PA: Lippincott Williams & Wilkins.

Reilly, M. (1962). Occupational therapy can be one of the greatest ideas of 20th century medicine. *American Journal of Occupational Therapy, 16*, 2–9.

Shannon, P. D. (1977). The derailment of occupational therapy. *American Journal of Occupational Therapy, 31*, 229–234.

abnormal psychology: A branch of psychology concerned with abnormal human behavior.

acetylcholine: A neurotransmitter that is especially important in transmitting signals between nerves and muscles.

active assisted range of motion (AAROM): Active range of motion that is bolstered by the help of another person (therapist).

active range of motion (AROM): The amount of movement an individual can accomplish at any given joint using his own muscle power, without help.

activity analysis: The analysis of an activity by breaking it down into its many constituent components.

activity of daily living (ADL): Any activity that is performed a on a daily basis by an individual. These include eating, dressing, and bathing.

agonist: The prime mover in a muscle group (e.g., the biceps muscle is the agonist for elbow flexion).

anatomy: The structure of an organism, especially the human body.

antagonist: A muscle (or group of muscles) that performs the opposite movement of the agonist (e.g., the triceps muscle is the antagonist of the biceps muscle because it extends the elbow).

anxiety disorder: A psychiatric condition that produces a profound and, often, unrealistic feeling of apprehension in an individual, impairing his ability to function adequately.

apraxia: The inability to perform purposeful movements or acts not due to motor, sensory, or coordination impairment.

ascending paralysis: Weakness or paralysis that is first seen in the legs and gradually moves upward toward the trunk and arms; this condition is typically seen in Guillain-Barré syndrome.

aspirate: To inhale a solid or liquid, such as food or water, into the lungs. If unresolved, aspiration pneumonia may occur.

assistive technology/devices: Any device or devices that can facilitate a person's independence in the performance of an occupation. Assistive technology can range from low-tech devices, such as neoprene foam used to build up the handle of a fork, to sophisticated computer-controlled environmental control systems for a quadriplegic.

ataxia/ataxic: A lack of coordination in voluntary movements typically caused by damage to the cerebellum.

athetoid: Involuntary slow, writhing muscle movements usually seen in certain types of cerebral palsy.

auditory hallucinations: Hearing sounds or voices in the absence of appropriate stimuli. Frequently seen in schizophrenia and mania, auditory hallucinations are much more common than visual hallucinations.

backward chaining: Teaching an activity backward in a step-by-step process, starting with the finished product and working in reverse until the first step is reached. Typically used to teach severely retarded individuals.

bariatrics: The field of medicine that focuses on the treatment and control of obesity and diseases associated with obesity.

battle fatigue: Negative physical and emotional responses to the effects of war (also called battle neurosis). Before World War II, this condition was known as shell shock. Today, it is known as post-traumatic stress disorder (PTSD) and is the result of any traumatic event, not just war.

behaviorism: A school of psychological theory that believes a person's behaviors are the result of environment, cause, and effect.

bipolar disorder: A psychiatric disorder that causes the patient to experience extreme mood swings, ranging from severe depression to a state of manic euphoria in which the patient has little or no impulse control. This is due to a chemical imbalance and is typically controlled by medication.

blindness: The severe decrease or total absence of vision.

blistering: The practice of applying solutions to the skin to cause blistering (a second-degree burn), meant to draw out infections or bad humors in the form of blood or pus.

bloodletting: Also known as bleeding. Incisions were made in a vein in order to drain a quantity of blood, in an attempt to restore the balance of bodily humors or to relieve tension and congestion in the arteries. This was not particularly effective; in fact, this practice led to the death of George Washington in an attempt to cure a throat infection.

body scheme: How an individual perceives her body in relation to the environment.

carpal tunnel syndrome (CTS): A condition in which the median nerve is trapped and compressed in the carpal tunnel formed by the wrist bones. This causes numbness and pain in the thumb, index, and middle fingers of the affected hand(s).

caseload: The total number of patients or clients seen by a therapist on a daily or weekly basis.

cataract: A clouding of the lens of the eye that impairs vision.

center of gravity (COG): The balance point at which the weight on all sides is equal. This is typically located just above the umbilicus (belly button).

cerebral palsy: A condition caused by brain damage that can occur before birth (prenatal), during the birthing process (perinatal), or at any point after birth (postnatal), up to the age of eight years old. This can cause both physical and cognitive irreversible impairments in the child.

certified occupational therapy assistant (COTA): An individual possessing a certificate or associate's degree in occupational therapy from a school accredited by the Accreditation Council for Occupational Therapy Education (ACOTE) and who has successfully passed the certification examination administered by the National Board for Certification in Occupational Therapy (NBCOT).

clinical reasoning: The skills that allow therapists to make judgements based on observation, knowledge, and experience.

cognition: High-level functions carried out by the human brain, including comprehension and use of speech, visual perception and construction, calculation ability, attention (information processing), memory, and executive functions such as planning, problem solving, and self-monitoring.

conditioned response: A response that has been learned by employing a specific stimulus.

contracture: A permanent shortening of a muscle and its corresponding joint, resulting in decreased range of motion.

contrast bath: The alternating use of hot and cold water to increase blood circulation to the hands or feet.

cryotherapy: The use of cold packs or cold water as a treatment modality.

deep pressure: The awareness of pressure at the level of bones, joints, and tendons.

deinstitutionalization: The process of removing the needy from residential facilities and placing them back in the community; reduction in the size of populations held in institutions by involuntary confinement, primarily mental hospitals and prisons. This movement began in the 1970s and was very successful in reducing the populations of mental hospitals.

degenerative joint disease (DJD): See **osteoarthritis.**

depression: A mental health disorder characterized by sadness, anger, and decreased biological drives and motivation. Depression is the most common mental health disorder in the world.

dermatome: A specific area of the body that is innervated by a specific sensory nerve.

developmental milestones: Abilities—such as turning over, sitting up, crawling, and walking—that children should achieve by a certain age to be considered within the norm of their peers. Failure to achieve these goals is indicative of developmental delay.

diagnostic honesty: A concept and tenet of hospice care in which all questions and concerns posed by the patient and his family regarding the outcome of the disease process will be answered honestly and openly, with no attempts to keep the information secret for the patient's own good.

diagnostic related group (DRG): One of 468 diagnosis categories based on age, gender, primary and secondary diagnoses, and intervention procedures that determine length of stay in a hospital and the amount of reimbursement received.

dopamine: A neurotransmitter formed in the *substantia nigra* in the brain. Lack of dopamine can cause clinical depression and is a significant cause of Parkinson's disease.

dressing stick: A device to help individuals who are unable to reach their lower body easily to don and remove underwear, pants, shoes, and socks.

dyad: Two individuals involved in a socially significant relationship (e.g., occupational therapist and client).

dynamometer: An instrument used to test hand-grip strength in both pounds and kilograms.

dysphagia: Difficulty swallowing, usually caused by brain damage or damage to the glossopharengeal nerve (cranial nerve IX).

dysphasia: A speech disorder in which a person's speech is impaired, accompanied by a lack of speech comprehension. The word comes from the Latin *dys-* (impairment) and the Greek *phasia* (speech).

Education for All Handicapped Children Act of 1975: An act passed by Congress in 1975 requiring that all children be given "free and appropriate" educational opportunities in the "least restrictive" environment. It was reauthorized in 1990 as the Individuals with Disabilities Education Act (PL 101–476); the most recent revision was PL 105–17 in 1997.

ego: The part of the psyche that maintains conscious contact with reality, and tempers the primitive impulses of the ego and the stern demands of the superego.

electrical muscle stimulation (EMS): Electrical stimulation to promote muscle tone and prevent atrophy.

electroconvulsive therapy (ECT): A treatment for certain psychiatric conditions in which an electric current is applied to the brain, causing a seizure designed to "reset" the brain and alleviate the psychiatric problems.

electrotherapy: The use of electricity to reduce edema and pain, and to facilitate muscle function.

ethics: The discipline dealing with what is good and bad, and with moral duty and obligation.

evaluate: To assess a client's abilities and disabilities. This typically includes physical, mental, and cognitive functioning, as well as the client's immediate environment.

evaluation, initial: The first meeting with, and assessment of, a new client.

exacerbation: To make or get worse.

facilitator: This person makes it easier for a group to get its work done, usually by way of nondirect leadership. The facilitator's role is one of assistance and guidance, not control.

fine motor: Pertaining to skills related to the use of the hands and fingers to perform delicate tasks such as buttoning, zipping, sewing, and so forth.

finger dynamometer: An instrument used to test the strength of the extrinsic and intrinsic hand muscles.

flaccid: Lacking muscle tone.

fluidotherapy: A modality that uses ground corn husks suspended in warm air to help reduce pain and increase range of motion.

forensic psychiatry: Aspect of psychiatry that deals with people who are incarcerated for a crime but are also mentally ill.

forward chaining: A method of teaching that involves starting with the initial steps of a task and continuing the task through to completion.

Freud, Sigmund: The "Father of Psychoanalysis." Freud believed that people's emotional problems are caused by internal battles between the id, ego, and superego. Although many of his theories are no longer relevant, he shaped the profession of modern psychiatry and coined many of the psychological terms used today.

functional electrical stimulation (FES): The application of low-level, computer-controlled electric current to the neuromuscular system, including paralyzed muscle, to enhance or produce functions such as walking or bike exercises.

gastroenterology: The study of diseases affecting the digestive tract.

gatekeeper: A member of a group (usually the leader) who controls what is allowed into the group system and may call for a change in the group's needs or abilities.

glaucoma: A symptomless condition of the eyes caused by increased intraocular pressure that, if untreated, can lead to blindness.

glucometer: A device that measures the amount of glucose (sugar) in an individual's blood. This is used daily by diabetics to help determine how much insulin is needed to maintain a normal blood glucose level.

goniometer: An instrument used to measure the movement of a joint.

graphesthesia: The ability to recognize numbers and words written on the skin without looking.

Great Society, the: A series of domestic initiatives introduced by President Lyndon B. Johnson in 1964. Among the programs instituted as part of this initiative were Medicare and Medicaid.

gross motor: Relating to the use of the larger muscle groups in the body to perform activities such as lifting, walking, swimming, and so forth.

group dynamics: The study of the interaction between members of a group and groups in general.

habit training: A treatment method involving a strict 24-hour regimen balancing work, self-care, play, rest, and sleep, designed to help psychiatric patients overcome or modify disorganized habits. It was first proposed by Adolf Meyer and was frequently used by Eleanor Clarke Slagle.

hospice: A concept, developed by Dame Cicely Saunders in England in 1968, that tends to the needs of the terminally ill and their families.

human growth and development: The dynamic process of growth and change in the human body and mind from prenatal development through old age and death.

hydrocollator: A device used to heat hot packs.

hyperglycemia: Too much blood glucose (sugar)—usually 126 milligrams per deciliter (mg/dL) or higher—which is usually an indicator of diabetes mellitus.

hypoglycemia: Too little blood glucose (sugar)—usually less than 60 milligrams per deciliter (mg/dL). This condition can result from too much insulin in the blood.

hypotonic/hypotonia: A condition of low muscle tone.

id: The part of the psyche that gives rise to basic impulses and drives.

inclusion: An educational concept designed to include children with disabilities in a regular classroom setting rather than segregate them into special schools or classrooms.

incontinence: The inability to control one's bladder or bowels.

Individualized Education Program (IEP): A written education plan for a school-aged child with disabilities, developed by a team of professionals (teachers, therapists, etc.) and the child's parents. IEPs are required under Public Law 94–142, the Individuals with Disabilities Education Act (IDEA).

Individuals with Disabilities Education Act of 1997 (IDEA): A federal law mandating that all children with disabilities have available to them a free, appropriate public education that emphasizes special education and related services designed to meet their unique needs and prepare them for employment and independent living.

instrumental activity of daily living (IADL): A more complex activity, not necessarily done every day, that is important to independent living. This includes preparing meals, doing housework, laundry, shopping, using transportation, managing money, using the telephone, and performing home maintenance.

insulin shock/insulin coma: The effect caused by an overdose of insulin, a decreased amount of food, or increased exercise. Symptoms include sweating, trembling, hunger, dizziness, moodiness, confusion, and numbness in the arms and hands. This condition is also referred to as an insulin reaction or hypoglycemia.

interest inventory: An instrument designed to determine what types of activities an individual enjoys or may be interested in trying.

internist: A doctor who specializes in internal medicine.

iontophoresis: The introduction of ions of soluble salts into tissues by direct current.

itinerant therapist: A traveling therapist who goes from place to place (usually among different schools within a school district).

joint protection: An educational process used by occupational therapists to help arthritic clients perform daily tasks in ways that put as little stress on their joints as possible.

Jung (pronounced yung), Carl: Swiss psychiatrist who founded analytical psychology. Though not the first to analyze dreams, his contributions to dream analysis are perhaps the most influential and certainly the most extensive. His approach to human psychology is unique, in that he placed primary emphasis on understanding the human psyche by means of exploring the world of dreams, art, mythology, world religion, and philosophy.

kinesiology: The study of movement.

kinesthesia: The sense of active movement.

leader: In a group setting, the leader (usually the therapist) is responsible for planning and running the group.

length of stay (LOS): In hospitals, mean length of stay is calculated by dividing the sum of inpatient days by the number of patients within the DRG category. Inpatient days are calculated by subtracting the day of admission from the day of discharge, so someone entering and leaving a hospital on the same day has a length of stay of zero.

light touch: Superficial touch on the skin.

long-term goal (LTG): A goal that focuses on the ultimate achievement of therapy. A long-term goal, once achieved, should lead to a client's discharge from therapy. The long-term goal is achieved by using numerous, smaller, short-term goals.

low vision: Also called partial sight. Sight that cannot be satisfactorily corrected with glasses, contacts, or surgery. Low vision usually results from an eye disease, such as glaucoma or macular degeneration. There are specialized optical and nonoptical devices that can enhance or improve visual ability in the low-vision patient. The selection of the proper device to be used is determined by a special low-vision eye examination.

macular degeneration: The loss of central vision in one or both eyes as a result of malfunctioning cone cells in the retina; "wet" (disciform) and "dry" (atrophic) are the two types. Also known as age-related macular degeneration (ARMD or AMD) and previously known as senile macular degeneration.

manic depression: See **bipolar disorder.**

Manual Muscle Test (MMT): A quasi-objective test of muscle strength in which the therapist asks the client to perform specific joint movements, either without or against gravity. The extent of movement, combined with the addition of gravity and other resistance, determines the muscle grade.

mastectomy: The surgical removal of a breast.

Medicaid: A jointly-funded, state and federal government insurance program that pays for medically necessary services. Medicaid pays for medical services for children and their caretakers, pregnant women, and people who are disabled, blind, or 65 years of age or older who can demonstrate a need through income and assets standards. In Illinois, Medicaid is administered by the Department of Public Aid. Medicaid funds physician, hospital, and long-term care.

Medicare: A federal insurance program providing a wide range of benefits to participating providers and suppliers. Medicare providers are patient care institutions such as hospitals, hospices, nursing homes, and home health agencies. Benefits are payable to most people over the age of 65, Social Security beneficiaries under the age of 65 who are entitled to disability benefits, and individuals needing renal dialysis or transplantation.

mental retardation: Impaired or incomplete mental development characterized by an IQ of 70 or lower and characterized by significant functional limitations in at least two of the following skills: communication, self-care, home living, social/interpersonal skills, use of community resources, self-direction, functional academic skills, work, leisure, health, and safety. Onset usually occurs before the age of 18. More than 200 specific causes of mental retardation have been identified.

moral treatment: An approach to treating the mentally ill with kindness and providing them with the means to care for themselves, rather than punishing them by chaining and imprisoning/institutionalizing them.

myelin: A fatty covering around nerve cells that helps to conduct nervous impulses. Myelin is destroyed by certain diseases—multiple sclerosis, for example—that cause difficulty in the smooth transmission of impulses.

neuroanatomy: The study of the structure and organization of the nervous system.

neurodevelopmental training (NDT): A form of neurological rehabilitation in which abnormal movement patterns are inhibited and, simultaneously, normal patterns are facilitated.

neurology: The study of the nervous system and its disorders.

neuromuscular junction: The synaptic site at which nerve endings meet the muscle tissue and nervous impulses are converted to muscle contractions.

neuroscience: The study of the function of the nervous system and the factors that influence its function.

objective: Information that can be effectively measured in such a way as to be adequately repeated by others, and that has subjectivity removed from the findings.

occupational history: An instrument used by occupational therapists to determine an individual's likes, dislikes, hopes, and aspirations. It is used to help the therapist view the individual as a person first and a medical condition second.

occupational therapist, registered (OTR): An individual who has completed a minimum of five years of training in an occupational therapy curriculum accredited by the Accreditation Council for Occupational Therapy Education (ACOTE) and who has successfully passed the registration examination administered by the National Board for Certification in Occupational Therapy (NBCOT).

orchiectomy: The surgical removal of a testicle.

orthotics: An external device applied to the body that is designed to immobilize or restrain injured tissues, align or correct deformity, or improve function.

osteoarthritis (OA): A form of arthritis involving the deterioration of the cartilage that cushions the ends of bones within joints. Also called degenerative arthritis, degenerative joint disease, or osteoarthrosis.

paradigm: An example or pattern that others may use as a guide; a model.

paraplegic: An individual who is unable to move from the chest down due to to a spinal cord injury at, or below, the thoracic level.

paresthesia: Abnormal sensations, such as burning, tingling, or a "pins and needles" feeling. Paresthesia may constitute the first group of symptoms of peripheral neuropathy, or it may be a limited drug side-effect that does not worsen with time.

Parkinson's disease: A progressive nervous disease occurring most often after the age of 50, associated with the destruction of brain cells that produce dopamine and characterized by muscular tremor, slowing of movement, partial facial paralysis, peculiarity of gait and posture, and weakness. Also called paralysis agitans, or shaking palsy.

passive range of motion (PROM): The range of motion that is performed by an external force, such as a therapist, moving a joint through its arc of movement. The person whose limb is being moved remains relaxed or passive.

Pavlov, Ivan: Russian physiologist known for his work with conditioned response whereby a stimulus can evoke a constant and predictable response. His famous experiment involved conditioning a dog to associate the ringing of a bell with food, which caused the dog to salivate each time he heard a bell ring, regardless of whether food was given or not.

perception: In psychology and the cognitive sciences, perception is the process of acquiring, interpreting, selecting, and organizing sensory information. Methods of studying perception range from biological or physiological approaches, through psychological approaches, to the often abstract "thought experiments" of mental philosophy.

peripheral nervous system (PNS): Nerves that conduct impulses outside the brain and spinal cord (i.e., outside the central nervous system [CNS]). The cell bodies of PNS nerves reside in the CNS, with their lengths extending out to peripheral parts of the body.

personality disorder: Any one of a group of psychiatric disorders characterized by an inability to relate to others due to rigid, inflexible, and maladaptive behavior patterns.

phantom limb: The illusion that a limb still exists after it has been amputated.

phantom pain: Pain that seems to originate in the portion of the limb that was removed.

physiatry: The branch of medicine that deals with restoring function to a person who has been disabled as a result of a disease, disorder, or injury.

physical agent modality (PAM): Any energy or material applied to a patient to relieve pain and improve function. Examples include heat, cold, ultraviolet, and ultrasound.

physiology: Physiology (in Greek, *physis* = nature and *logos* = word) is the study of the mechanical, physical, and biochemical functions of living organisms.

plaque: Patchy area of inflammation, demyelination, and sclerosis in the CNS that is characteristic of multiple sclerosis damage.

polio: A viral disease that causes muscular paralysis. Until the advent of the polio vaccine in the 1950s, polio was a cause of great concern and disability in the United States. Today, it is extremely rare.

praxis: The ability to plan and perform purposeful movements.

prefrontal lobotomy: The surgical method of severing the frontal cortex from the rest of the brain as a means of making the patient more compliant. This procedure was used from the 1930s through the 1950s but is no longer performed.

primary care physician (PCP): A "generalist" such as a family practitioner, pediatrician, internist, or obstetrician. In a managed care organization, a primary care physician is accountable for the total health services of enrollees, including referrals, procedures, and hospitalization.

private pay: Out-of-pocket payment for occupational therapy services with no third party payment involved.

proprioception: The ability to sense the position of the limbs and their movements with the eyes closed.

prospective payment system (PPS): A lump-sum system of reimbursement for health care services based on diagnoses.

prosthetics: Any device that replaces a lost or missing body part. Prosthetics can include arms, legs, breasts, testicles, eyes, and teeth. Prosthetics can be used for function, cosmetics, or both.

psychiatry: The medical specialty concerned with the origin, diagnosis, prevention, and treatment of mental disorders. Psychiatrists must obtain a medical degree and spend four years or more in approved residency training. They must also be licensed by their state in order to practice. As physicians, psychiatrists are the only mental health professionals licensed to prescribe medication.

purging: Inducing vomit in order to obtain a balance of bodily humors, or administering a laxative such as castor oil to promote bowel movements.

quadriplegia: A condition caused by damage to the spinal cord at the cervical spine or the brain. The injury causes the victim to lose either total or partial use of the arms and legs. The condition is also termed tetraplegia; both terms mean "paralysis of four limbs."

range of motion (ROM): The ability of a joint to go through all its normal movements. Range-of-motion exercises help increase or maintain flexibility and movement in muscles, tendons, ligaments, and joints.

referral: An official request for occupational therapy services, usually made by a physician.

remission: A period of time during which all or some of the symptoms of a disease have disappeared or decreased in severity. Remission may occur spontaneously or as a result of medical treatment.

repetitive stress injury: An occupational overuse syndrome affecting muscles, tendons, and nerves in the arms and upper back. It occurs when muscles in these areas are kept tense for very long periods of time, due to poor posture or repetitive motions.

resting tremor: Shaking that occurs in a relaxed limb. It usually stops when a voluntary movement of the affected limb is made.

rheumatoid arthritis: An autoimmune disease that causes chronic inflammation of the joints, the tissue around the joints, and other organs in the body. Because it can affect multiple organs, rheumatoid arthritis is a systemic illness and is sometimes called rheumatoid disease.

rocker knife: A knife with a curved blade that allows a person to use the blade as a fulcrum to cut food by rocking the knife rather than sawing.

Rogers, Carl: An American psychologist who developed the client-centered approach to psychotherapy.

schizophrenia: A psychiatric condition in which the patient experiences a disassociation between sensory input, thoughts, feelings, and emotions. Schizophrenics frequently experience auditory hallucinations.

scoliosis: A lateral (sideways) curvature of the spine associated with rotation, so that, in the thoracic spine, the ribs on the convex side are placed backward. Some degree of spinal asymmetry is common, with 25% of the population experiencing this in childhood. Curves of over 20° occur in one to two of every thousand boys and four to five of every thousand girls. Sixty-five percent of all cases are idiopathic (cause is not known). Most scoliosis occurs in girls at the start of adolescence.

screening: A brief, informal assessment of a person's possible need for occupational therapy services. A screening is typically not reimbursed by third party payers.

sensory integration: The neurological process of organizing and processing, or perceiving sensations for use.

shell shock: The World War I version of battle fatigue/battle neurosis.

short-term goal (STG): A goal necessary to achieve an ultimate long-term goal and eventually discharge the client from therapy.

side neglect: A perceptual impairment following a brain injury, such as a stroke, in which the individual is unaware of one side of his body and tends to neglect that side during all activities.

Skinner, B. F.: The "Father of Operant Conditioning," a form of psychology that emphasized the control of behavior through a series of conditioned responses.

sock aid: One of many devices that enables an individual to easily don socks with little or no bending involved.

spasticity/spastic: An involuntary increase in muscle tone (tension) that occurs following injury to the brain or spinal cord, causing the muscles to resist being moved. Characteristics may include an increase in deep tendon reflexes, resistance to passive stretches, clasp-knife phenomenon, and clonus.

stereognosis: The ability to identify an object by its shape.

stress loading: Applying gradually increased pressure and duration of pressure to a limb affected by complex regional pain syndrome in an effort to decrease edema and pain.

superego: The part of the psyche that acts as the parental control over the subconscious id and ego.

superficial heating agent (SHA): A heating agent, such as a hot pack, that is applied to the skin and acts upon superficial layers of tissue.

superficial pain: Pain that can be felt on the skin, such as a sunburn, a slap on the face, or a pin prick.

superficial physical agent modality (SPAM): An agent, such as a cold pack, that is applied to the skin for therapeutic purposes.

synergist: A muscle (or group of muscles) that acts together with an agonist or antagonist to facilitate a particular movement.

tactile: Pertaining to the sense of touch.

Temporal Adaptation Assessment: An assessment of how a person uses time during the course of a day.

tenodesis splint: A dynamic (moving) orthotic device or splint that allows the user to pick up and release objects with limited muscular control of a hand. Frequently used by quadriplegics.

therapeutic ultrasound: An electrical modality that transmits a sound wave through an applicator, into the skin, and to the soft tissue in order to heat the local area for relaxing the injured tissue or dispersing edema.

thermal sensations: Hot and cold.

third party payer: A person or agency that pays for part or all of an individual's medical expenses. Examples include Blue Cross/Blue Shield and Medicare.

transfer board: A flat board with beveled edges that is highly sanded, polished, and shellacked, in order to allow an individual to sit on it and push or slide across it from one point to another, without having to stand. Sometimes called a sliding board, it serves as a bridge to help an individual safely transfer from one point to another.

transcutaneous electric nerve stimulation (TENS): A nonaddictive and noninvasive method of pain control that applies electric impulses to nerve endings via electrodes that are attached to a stimulator by flexible wires and placed on the skin. The electric impulses block the transmission of pain signals to the brain.

traumatic brain injury (TBI): An insult to the brain, caused by an external physical force, that may produce a diminished or altered state of consciousness that results in an impairment of cognitive abilities or physical functioning and/or a disturbance of behavioral or emotional functioning.

treatment plan: A plan established by the therapist, in conjunction with the client, that lays out how the treatment process will proceed, the types of intervention proposed, and all short- and long-term goals.

trephining: The removal of a circular piece of bone, usually from the skull. This was originally practiced to alleviate mental illness by boring a hole in the skull to release evil spirits.

two-point discrimination: The ability to detect two separate and distinct points applied to the skin simultaneously at varying distances.

ultrasound: See **therapeutic ultrasound**.

vascular dementia: A common cause of memory loss or dementia in older people, this is due to the blockage of the small arteries that supply the brain with oxygen, leading to very small strokes that can cause progressive brain damage.

vestibular/vestibular system: Pertaining to the vestibular system in the middle ear and the brain, which senses movements of the head. Disorders of the vestibular system can lead to dizziness, poor regulation of postural muscle tone, and the inability to detect quick movements of the head.

wellness: The opposite of illness; a proactive method to maintain health and avoid disease.

workers' compensation insurance: Insurance paid to individuals who are temporarily unable to work due to a job-related injury; the insurance continues until the individual recovers or finds another line of work.

INDEX

Note: Page numbers in *italic* type indicate figures or illustrations.

A

Abnormal psychology, 48
Accreditation Council for Occupational
  Therapy Education (ACOTE), 44
Acetylcholine, 150–151
Acknowledgement, of clients, 60
Active assisted range of motion, 87
Active range of motion, 87
Activities, appropriateness of
  therapeutic, 100
Activities of daily living (ADLs), *31*, 80, 96
Activity analysis, 50–51
Activity therapists, 65, 77–78
Adaptive equipment. *See* Assistive
  technology
ADHD. *See* Attention-deficit hyperactivity
  disorder
Agonists, 47
AIDS, 114, 148, *149*
Alzheimer's disease, 120–121
American Occupational Therapy
  Association (AOTA), 4–6, 22, *25*,
  26, 53
American Psychiatric Association, 128
Amputations, 133–134
Amyotrophic lateral sclerosis (ALS), 133
Anatomy, 47
Anesthesia, 92
Anger management training, 64, 169
Anorexia nervosa, 124
Antagonists, 47
Anxiety disorders, 48, 121
Apraxia, 96
Arthritis, 134–136
Ascending paralysis, 146
Asperger's syndrome (AS), 108
Aspiration, 79
Assistive technology, 52, 78, 135
Ataxic cerebral palsy, 110
Athetoid cerebral palsy, 110
Attention-deficit hyperactivity disorder
  (ADHD), 80, 107–108
Auditory hallucinations, 128
Autism spectrum disorders (ASD),
  108–109
Ayres, Jean, *25*, 118

B

Backward chaining, 112
Bariatrics, 136
Barton, George Edward, 21, 22, 39
Basket weaving, 22, 51
Battle fatigue, 22
Beck Depression Inventory, *127*
Becker muscular dystrophy, 116
Behaviorism, 48
Bethlehem (Bedlam) Hospital,
  London, 18
Bible, 16
Bipolar disorder, 48, 127–128
Blindness, 155
Blistering, 17
Bloodletting, 17, *18*
Body language, 60
Body scheme, 96
Bonder, B. R., 129
Boredom, 6
Boutonniere deformity, *135*
Bracciano, A., 55
Brinkman, R., 83
Brown, J. D., 125
Bulimia nervosa, 124
Burke, Anne, 132
Burn injury classification, *137*
Burnout, 13
Burns, 136–137

C

Cancer, 109, 137–138
Cardiovascular disease, 138
Caregivers, interviews of, 85–86, *87*
Carpal tunnel syndrome (CTS), 66, 139,
  165–166
Caseloads, 82
Cataracts, 155, 156
Cawood, L. T., 30
Center of gravity, 170
Centers for Disease Control
  (CDC), *149*
Cerebral palsy, 109–110
Cerebrovascular accident, 140–141
Certified nurse aides, health care team
  role of, 75–76

196